THE HANDBOOK OF HOLISTIC

HEALING

Healing The Body Naturally

by

Dr. Earendil M. Spindelilus D.N.M., M.H., C.R., PSc.D

THE HANDBOOK OF HOLISTIC HEALING

COPYRIGHT © 2020 BY EARENDIL M. SPINDELILUS

ALL RIGHTS RESERVED.

PUBLISHED BY TREE OF LIFE HOLISTIC WELLNESS CENTER

COVER ART BY EARENDIL AND PEGGY SPINDELILUS

NO PART OF THIS BOOK MAY BE REPRODUCED IN ANY WRITTEN, ELECTRONIC, RECORDING OR PHOTOGRAPHING WITHOUT WRITTEN PERMISSION OF THE PUBLISHER OR AUTHOR.

FIRST EDITION. - **ISBN** - 9798605358756

DISCLAIMER

THIS BOOK IS INTENDED TO PROVIDE INFORMATION ON THE SUBJECT OF TREATING A WIDE VARIETY OF CONDITIONS AND ILLNESSES AT HOME WITH ALTERNATIVE METHODS. THIS INFORMATION PRESENTED IS NOT INTENDED AS A SUBSTITUTE FOR MEDICAL TRAINING OR ADVICE, BUT EVERY EFFORT HAS BEEN MADE TO ENSURE ACCURACY.

THE BOOK IS SOLD WITH THE UNDERSTANDING THAT THE PUBLISHER AND AUTHOR ARE NOT LIABLE FOR ANY MISCONCEPTION OR MISUSE OF THE INFORMATION PROVIDED AND SHALL HAVE NEITHER LIABILITY NOR RESPONSIBILITY TO ANY PERSON OR ENTITY WITH RESPECT TO ANY LOSS, DAMAGE OR INJURY CAUSED OR ALLEGED TO BE CAUSED DIRECTLY OR INDIRECTLY BY THE SAID INFORMATION.

DEDICATION

To my wife and best friend Peggy, who has stood beside me and put up with all of my time spent getting one degree or certification after another.

To Waya and Sinde, our furry children who love us unconditionally

I would also like to express my gratitude for all of the patients who have taught me so much about how to be a doctor.

Not all doctors are healers and not all healers are doctors.

Table of Contents

DEDICATION..3

LIST OF FIGURES..10

PART 1 – A COMPLETE BODY REPAIR

CHAPTER 1 INTRODUCTION..12

CHAPTER 2 CANDIDA – THE GREAT MIMICKER................................17

2.1 What is Candida?...17

2.2 Causes of Candida...23

2.3 Symptoms of Candida and related diseases...25

2.4 Current methods of diagnosis..33

2.5 Conventional methods of treatment...35

2.6 Holistic treatment – The Candida Cleanse..37

CHAPTER 3 PARASITES...49

3.1 What are parasites and how common are they?......................................49

3.2 Causes of parasites..55

3.3 Symptoms of parasites and related diseases...56

3.4 Current methods of diagnosis..58

3.5 Conventional methods of treatment...59

3.6 Holistic treatment – The Parasite Cleanse...61

CHAPTER 4 HEAVY METAL TOXICITY..65

4.1 What are heavy metals?...65

4.2 Causes of heavy metal toxicity……………………………………………………...67

4.3 Symptoms of heavy metal toxicity and related diseases……………………….....69

4.4 Current methods of diagnosis……………………………………………………...71

4.5 Conventional methods of treatment……………………………………………….72

4.6 Holistic treatment – The Heavy Metal Cleanse……………………………….......74

CHAPTER 5 HOW TO PREVENT THEIR RE-OCCURRENCE……………………..81

5.1 Diet as a major factor……………………………………………………………....81

5.2 Lifestyle choices……………………………………………………………………87

PART 2 – HOLISTIC FIRST-AID

CHAPTER 6 INTRODUCTION……………………………………………………..91

CHAPTER 7 BASIC FIRST-AID……………………………………………………94

7.1 Burns………………………………………………………………………………..94

7.2 Rashes……………………………………………………………………………..106

7.3 Bites and Stings…………………………………………………………………...115

7.4 Lice………………………………………………………………………………..124

7.5 Warts………………………………………………………………………………126

7.6 Abrasions/bruises…………………………………………………………………129

CHAPTER 8 INTERMEDIATE FIRST-AID………………………………………131

8.1 Ear Infections……………………………………………………………………..131

8.2 Dental ……………………………………………………………………………..135

8.3 Infections………………………………………………………………………….139

8.4 Allergic Reactions……………………..…………………………......144

8.5 Bleeding – Minor………………..…………………………….…...150

8.6 Eye Injuries and Infections……………………………....……...155

CHAPTER 9 ADVANCED……………………...………………....……159

9.1 Major Bleeding/Shock/Deep Cuts and Wounds………………..…...159

9.2 Poisoning………………………………………………………...166

9.3 Broken Bones………………………………………………..…...175

9.4 Heart attack/Stroke……………………………………………..…...179

9.5 Pain Management………………………………………………...183

CHAPTER 10 A SAMPLE FIRST-AID KIT……………………………191

10.1 First Aid Kit Supplies……………………………………….....191

10.2 How to make your own medications…………………………...194

PART 3 – A HOLISTIC APPROACH TO CURING LYME DISEASE

CHAPTER 11 INTRODUCTION…………………………………….199

11.1 What is Lyme disease?..202

11.2 Common Symptoms…..204

11.3 A history of misdiagnosis and misinformation........................207

11.4 Current methods of diagnosis…..209

11.5 Current methods of treatment….......................................211

CHAPTER 12 HOLISTIC PROTOCOLS…………………………….217

12.1 My protocols to date…...228

12.2 Candida Cleanse..229

12.3 Case Histories..238

CHAPTER 13 COMPLIMENTARY RESULTS COMPARED TO CONVENTIONAL
....242.

REFERENCES..244

PART 4 – CASE HISTORIES FROM A SUCCESSFUL NATUROPATHIC CLINIC

INTRODUCTION..249

CHAPTER 14 ACCIDENTS...253

14.1 PEGGY – KNIVES...253

14.2 PEGGY – BURNS..255

14.3 BOB – GANGRENE..256

CHAPTER 15 CHILDREN..263

15.1 JILL – PREGNANCY..263

15.2 JANE – PREGNANCY..266

15.3 MARK – IMPOTENT..267

15.4 "CUB" - SEVERE BRONCHITIS..268

15.5 JOHN – APPENDICITIS..269

15.6 MULTIPLE AUTISM CASES...270

15.7 LISA - MORBID OBESITY AND PREGNANCY....................................271

15.8 JOHNNY - ALMOST FATAL ANEMIA – AGE 21 MONTHS.................273

CHAPTER 16 LUNG ISSUES...275

16.1 WILLIAM – COPD..275

16.2 PAUL – TUBERCULOSIS..276

16.3 STEVE – CHRONIC PNEUMONIA/BRONCHITIS..................277

CHAPTER 17 CHRONIC..278

17.1 Ruth – Lyme Disease...278

17.2 Peggy – 92 prescription pills a week..280

17.3 Christine – High Blood Pressure...282

17.4 Susan – High Cholesterol/Triglycerides.....................................283

17.5 Jack – Near-Sighted..284

17.6 Virgil – Shingles and Heart Blockage...285

17.7 Betsy – Heavy metal toxicity..287

CHAPTER 18 INCURABLES..290

18.1 LILLY – UTECAREA...290

18.2 BETTY – MULTIPLE SCLEROSIS...292

18.3 MATTHEW – SIGMOID CANCER..294

18.4 STACY – POLYCYSTIC OVARIAN SYNDROME..................296

18.5 JAMES – PSORIASIS/GENETIC ISSUES................................298

18.6 ROBERT – TYPE 1 DIABETES...301

18.7 NANCY – MYASTHENIA GRAVIS..303

18.8 CATHY – EPSTEIN BARR..*306*

18.9 CAROL – HYSTERECTOMY AT AGE 27...............................*307*

18.10 SAMUEL – CHRONIC SYSTEM WIDE BODY RASH……………...………..*309*

18.11 KIM – INOPERABLE COLON/APPENDIX CANCER………………………..*311*

BONUS SECTION – ANIMAL FIRST-AID……………………………………..…314

ABOUT THE AUTHOR……………………………………...………………....323

LIST OF FIGURES

Figure 1. Stages of growth..201

Figure 2. Lyme tick on the march...203

Figure 3. Lyme rash examples..206

Figure 4. Lyme facts...208

Figure 5. Types of antibiotics used on conventional treatments........................212

Figure 6. Medication schedule for candida cleanse...231

PART ONE – A COMPLETE BODY REPAIR

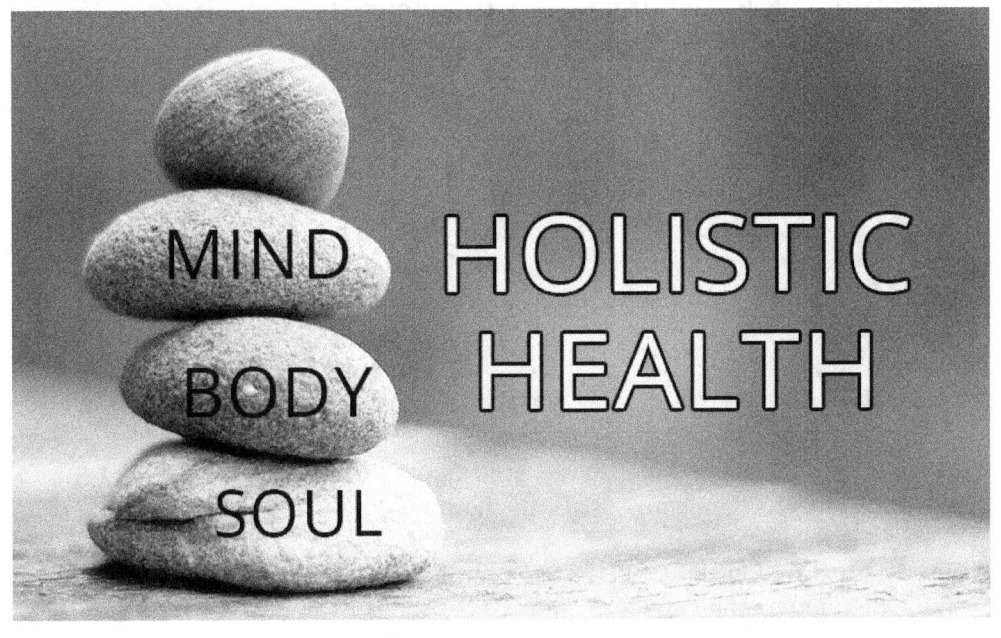

CHAPTER 1

Introduction

"Over 90% of all human diseases start in bowels"
Dr. John R. Christopher

Throughout my 20+ years of practice one of the most frustrating complaints I hear from new patients is the lack of a proper diagnosis. For most, they have spent years going from one doctor to another, sometimes trying both conventional and alternative methods, to no avail. They come to the clinic sad, angry, frustrated and bitter at the medical community and have little hope remaining. This is the common attitude I am faced with each day.

I certainly do understand how they feel and I can empathize with them. My dad tried for years to get a diagnose for his chronic pulmonary issues. He was diagnosed with congestive heart failure, bronchitis, etc. In the end, he passed away from simple pneumonia due to a string of doctors not taking the time to figure out what was happening inside his body.

A survey was done in the United States by the AMA on how long can a doctor spend with their patients before they begin to lose money. The results were shocking. The national average was 6 minutes. Many reasons were given. Some complained of too many patients in a day. Many doctors will see up to 30 or more patients a day. Proper attention to patients with this schedule is pretty much unattainable. I have made it a point to spend no less than 30 minutes with each one.

Yes, this causes me to see less patients in the day, but each in turn gets a higher quality of attention and I am better able to do a proper intake and discuss their issues. Other reasons were also given. Another example was the cost of our overhead as a doctor. I have found this can also be misleading. I have the same insurance as most doctors in California and I actually have a higher overhead as we are not just a private practice with an office and a receptionist but a full clinic. And yet, I can still spend the time with each patient as needed. The reason for this is sometimes as simple as the overhead of the doctor's lifestyle itself.

So, it is not unusual to find patients coming into the clinic stating their other doctors simply did not take the time to properly diagnosis their problems. What is also lacking is a proper application of diagnostic procedures. In medical school you learn about a variety of medical procedures and protocols commonly used to diagnosis a patient's presenting complaints. We learn about doing a proper intake when the patient first arrives at the clinic. We do vitals, urinalysis, blood work, scans, etc. All of these are fine and I do take advantage of each of these valuable tools. What is often missing is the education required to investigate the root cause.

Part of the medical code of ethics behind Naturopathic Medicine is to get to the root cause of the condition, not to simply treat the symptoms, This is one of the great powers of the Naturopathic profession, if properly applied. Unfortunately, even in the Naturopathic community, more and more of them are forgetting their lessons in chronic illness diagnosis and are finding it more profitable to simply treat the symptoms. I have also had occasions where an M.D. would come up to me when I was working in their hospitals and would complain about the lack of education they had received in medical school for diagnosing the root cause of chronic diseases. Some of them even went back to school years later to start their certification in Naturopathic Medicine. It is definitely a good start.

Again, after so many years of practice what have I discovered about the root causes among so many patients today in western civilization? In this, I have discovered the accuracy of the old adage, *"Life is very simple, it is ourselves who complicate it"*.

Common knowledge today states that as a species, humans are rarely living a natural life and the lifestyle choices they make are usually in conflict with our nature. Fast foods comprise the greater content of most diets in America and rarely do they eat anything living. Sadly, nutritional education is becoming less and less common in schools today and most doctors receive little to no nutritional education in medical school, against federal mandates from the 1990s.

It is in part because of this lack of knowledge on the doctor's behalf that illness continues to spread in the World's wealthiest nations. According to Clinic Compare out of Britain, they analyzed 179 countries based on information from the World Health Organization. America is the only non-European country to make the top 10 unhealthiest on the list, having the ninth highest rate of obesity in the world — 35% of the adult population is classified as dangerously overweight. It is considered the sickest nation in the developed World. As well as from other studies the results surprised even the researchers. To their alarm, they said, they found a "strikingly consistent and pervasive" pattern of poorer health at all stages of life, from infancy to childhood to adolescence to young adulthood to middle and old age. Compared to people in other developed nations, Americans die far more often from injuries and homicides. We suffer more deaths from alcohol and other drugs, and endure some of the worst rates of heart disease, lung disease, obesity, and diabetes. Among the most striking of the findings are that, among the countries studied, the U.S. has:

• The highest rate of death by violence, by a stunning margin
• The highest rate of death by car accident, also dramatically so
• The highest chance that a child will die before age 5
• The second-highest rate of death by coronary heart disease
• The second-highest rate of death by lung disease
• The highest teen pregnancy rate
• The highest rate of women dying due to complications of pregnancy and childbirth

According to Pure Wellness out of the U.K., the United States has one of the worst diets in the World. As stated on their website: "…where every portion of food or drink can be 'super-sized'. This is the world of plenty! But where did it all go wrong for this nation? According to the documentary, it all started back in 1971 where President Nixon was hopeful for a re-election. Many Americans at the time were very unhappy about the high cost of food. So to get the price down, Nixon encouraged farmers to mass produce crops……and one in particular—corn! This process created a new product called high fructose corn syrup (HFCS)—A cheap sugar sweetener that can be found in thousands of food products today. However, it didn't just stay in America. This processed product spread like wild fire to other countries with similar dieting problems."

Stress levels are also on the rise. A recent report shows America to be among the most stressed out nations on Earth. People are becoming more and more disconnected from the natural world and spending their lives in an environment devoid of trees, grass and open, quiet spaces. According to the website **Gostress.,com**:

STRESS RELATED FACTS AND STATISTICS

- The Stress in America survey results show that adults continue to report high levels of stress and many report that their stress has increased over the past year – *American Psychological Association*.

- 75% of adults reported experiencing moderate to high levels of stress in the past month and nearly half reported that their stress has increased in the past year – *American Psychological Association*.

- Approximately 1 out of 75 people may experience panic disorder – *National Institutes of Mental Health*.

- Stress is a top health concern for U.S. teens between 9th and 12th grade, psychologists say that if they don't learn healthy ways to manage that stress now, it could have serious long-term health implications – *American Psychological Association*.

- 80% of workers feel stress on the job and nearly half say they need help in learning how to manage stress. And 42% say their co-workers need such help – *American Institute of Stress*.

- Stress levels in the workplace are rising with 6 in 10 workers in major global economies experiencing increased workplace stress. With China (86%) having the highest rise in workplace stress – *The Regus Group*

- Alarmingly 91% of adult Australians feel stress in at least one important area of their lives. Almost 50% feel very stressed about one part of their life – *Lifeline Australia*.

As can be seen from the above statistics, America and most of the western world is in a mess, health speaking. Combine this with a lack of education in Western Medicine for diagnosing chronic disease and you have a very frustrated culture with the medical community. But, there is good news. As stated earlier about Life actually being very simple, so often is the case, the cause can also be very simple. Enter, the root cause of most conditions … **candida, parasites and heavy metal toxicity**.

Within this book I will cover each of these topics in detail, describing what they are, the causes, how to diagnose, conditions caused by them, conventional treatments and how to successfully treat holistically.

CHAPTER 2

CANDIDA – THE GREAT MIMICKER

2.1 What is Candida

As reported by the CDC, *"Candidemia is one of the most common bloodstream infections in the United States."* Research from Rice University shows that **70 percent of all people have Candida, a systemic fungal infection, in their bodies.**[1] According to the molecular biologists at Rice University, Candida is common in humans and is often found in colonies in their intestines, mouths, or on their skin. When researchers delved deeper into how *Candida albicans* moved throughout the body, with findings published in the journal *PLOS One*, they noted that the "remarkable pathogen" Candida can cause infection in the body that is both superficial and systemic by penetrating epithelial barriers.

Definition of a Candida Overgrowth

The perforated bowel is referred to as Leaky Gut Syndrome. This condition also allows undigested protein to enter the bloodstream. These proteins are foreign to the immune system and are therefore attacked. The immune system remembers these protein invaders and reacts like an allergy each time you consume them. This opens up the possibility of eventually making you allergic to every food you eat.

Since yeast overgrowth can cause symptoms mimicking many diseases, misdiagnosis is common and yeast overgrowth remains undetected allowing it to further colonize, thus creating more side effects and ill health. Many people have suffered for decades going from doctor to doctor, therapy to therapy and eventually being prescribed anti-depressants from doctors who are incapable of a proper diagnosis, as they determine that it is in the head of the patients. This incompetence on the part of modern medicine hopefully leads these unfortunate patients to alternative therapy.

Most alternative therapy focuses on killing off the yeast and providing the body with the probiotics. These therapies fail to correct the damaged intestinal tract which allows the yeast condition to return.

According to the website **candidaplan.com:**

The human digestive tract is said to contain some 100 trillion cells compared to about only 10 trillion human cells in the body. This particular arrangement has led to man being classified as a "super-organism," whose health is directly related to the function of the thousands of species of micro-organisms that make up the 100 trillion cells in the intestinal tract. For years, research suggested that there were 400-500 species that made up this microbial population. Recent advances in research have now put that number at anywhere from 3,300 to 5,700 or more, to upwards of 30,000 species. The intestinal tract houses what has been called "the densest ecosystem on the planet," and is approximately 25-28 ft long. The surface area of the intestinal tract measures approximately 200 square meters, roughly the size of a tennis court.

The widespread use of antibiotics, which induce neutropenia, an abnormally low number of neutrophils (white blood cells), and immune system suppression is commonly attributed by science to be the most consistent cause of systemic Candida. Corticosteroids suppress immune system function. Intestinal homeostasis is critical for human health. Candida has been shown to be capable of causing systemic immuno-suppression via its cell wall proteins, TLR2-mediated IL-10 release, protease cleaving of leukocyte integrin CD11/CD18, and intracellular components. Candida can also manipulate inflammatory responses as needed and inflammatory responses can have systemic effects.

On top of everything else it can do, Candida has the ability to destroy immune cells, hide from the immune system, adapt to the inner environment of immune cells, resist and suppress ROI and NO production of immune cells, destroy binding sites and receptors of immune cells, manipulate immune responses, and affect immune cell structure.

With all of the above in mind, it is easy to see why so many Americans have a compromised immune system and why Candida leads the charge as one of the most common root causes for most disorders.

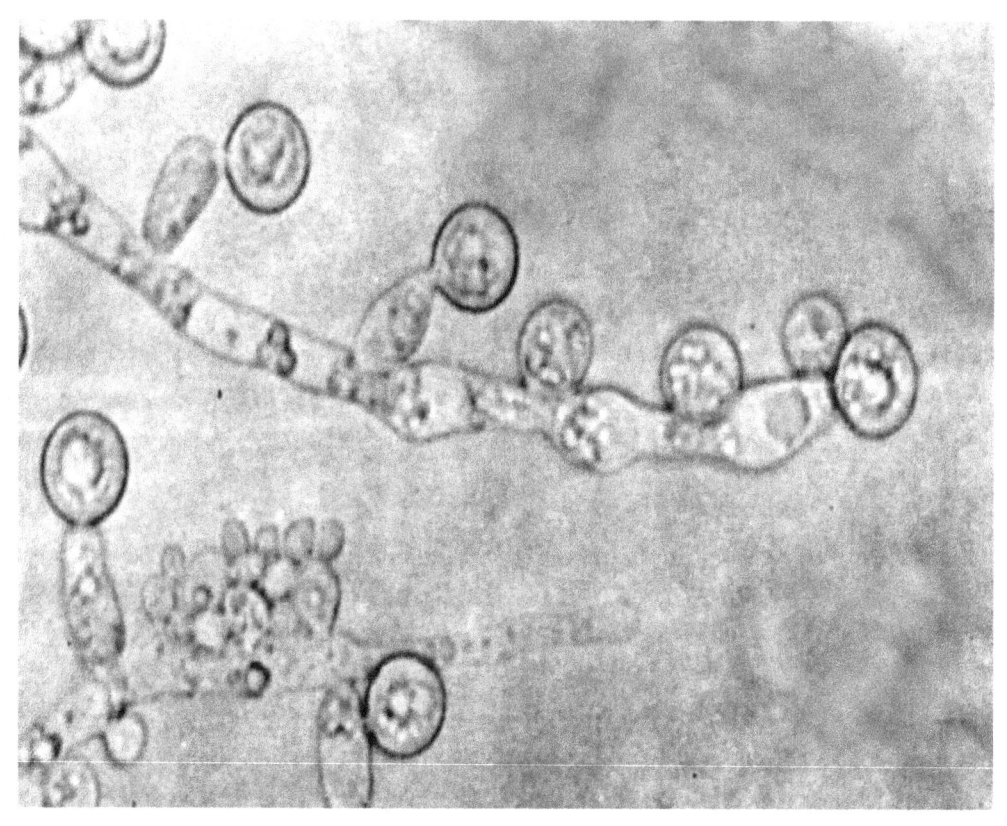

Candida Albicans

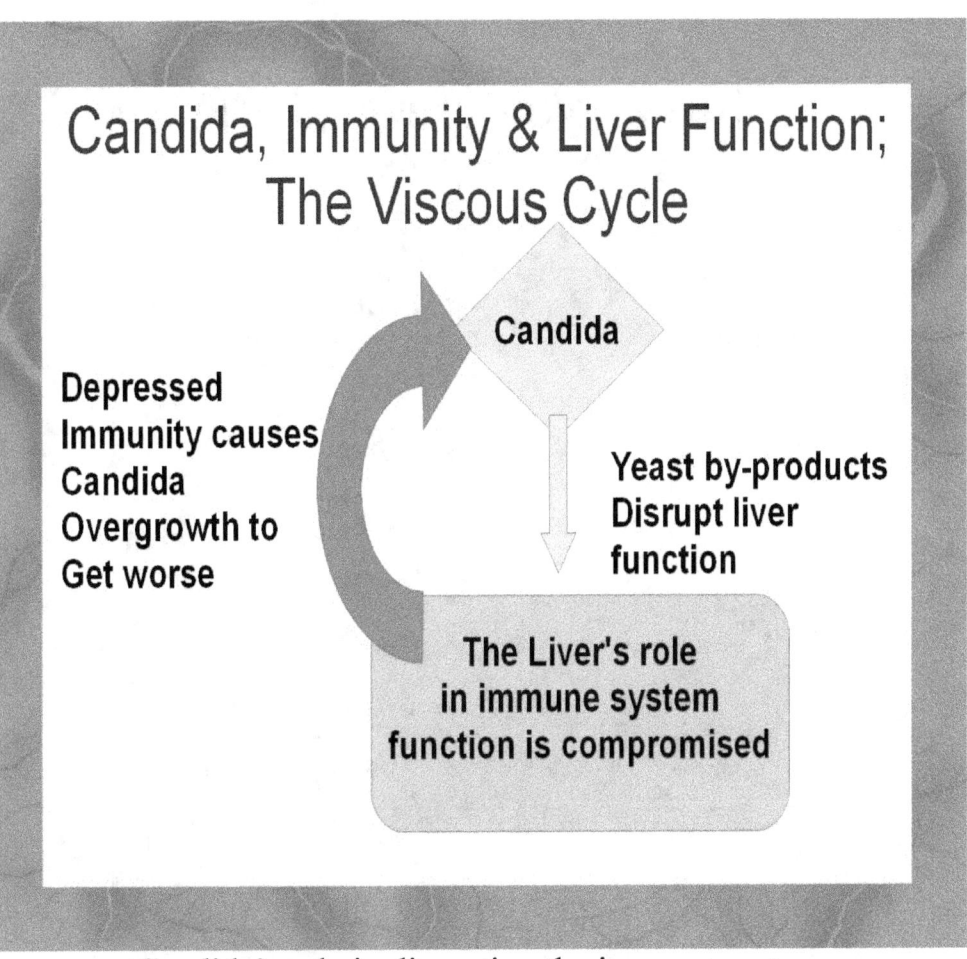

Candida's role in disrupting the immune system

The Candida Growth Cycle

- Overuse & Misuse of Prescription Antibiotics/Steroids
- Wipes Out Good Bacteria "Soldiers"
- Candida Multiplies
- "Leaky Gut" Releases Toxins Back into System
- Weakens Immune System/ADHD & Hyperactivity
- Re-Occuring
- Infection/Illness

Growth is Encouraged & Proliferated by Standard American Diet (simple carbs, sugars, dairy, poultry & beef antibiotics)

Candida's Growth Cycle

2.2 Causes of Candida

As common as this condition is, there are a few easily avoided causes for us to be aware of and lifestyle changes can aid us in eliminating the threat. Following is a list of some of the causes:

1.) A high sugar diet – processed sugars and carbs.

2.) Antibiotics – The number one cause.

3.) Chronic stress.

4.) Birth control pill

5.) Mercury in dental fillings.

6.) Various other chemical exposures found in products and the environment.

7.) Diabetes.

8.) Excessive alcohol use.

9.) Other heavy metal toxicity such as copper, nickel, lead, often found in metal implants.

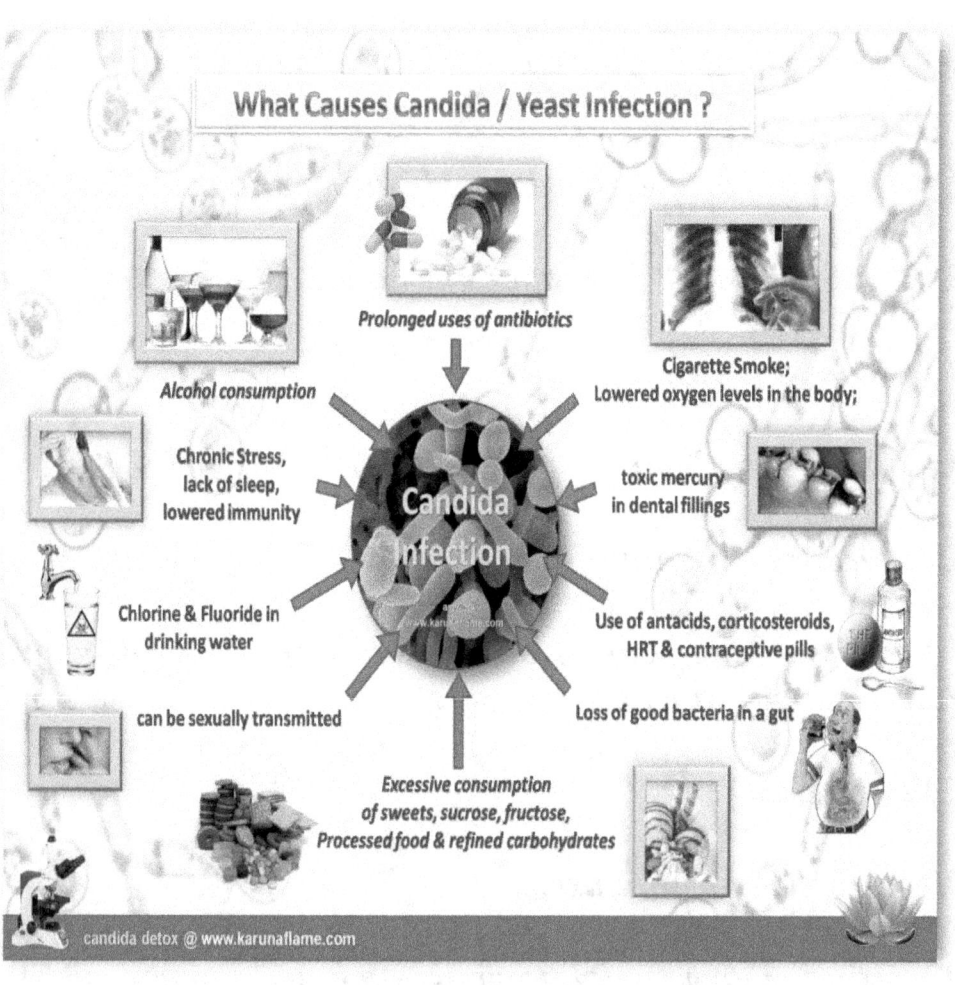

Causes of Candida

2.3 Symptoms of Candida and related diseases

Called The Great Imitator (along with Lyme), this disease is one of the great mimickers as it can appear as dozens of others conditions and is therefore routinely misdiagnosed. Following is a partial list of symptoms:

Please note these common Candida symptoms are also associated with many other disorders:

- **Bad breath**
- **Bloating, belching, intestinal gas, and/or abdominal pain**
- **Constipation or diarrhea**
- **Endometriosis or infertility**
- **Fatigue and chronic fatigue**
- **Frequent mood swings**
- **Impotence**
- **Insomnia**
- **Loss of sexual desire or feeling**
- **Muscle aches, weakness, or paralysis**
- **Pain and/or swelling in joints**
- **Poor memory, foggy thinking, or feeling "spacey"**
- **Prostatitis**

- **Troublesome vaginal itching, burning, or discharge**

  CANDIDA RELATED DISEASE (Just a few, there are many more)

- **Celiac Disease**
- **Leaky Gut Syndrome**
- **Crohn's Disease**
- **Thrush**
- **Autism**
- **Irritable Bowel Syndrome**
- **Chronic Sinusitis**
- **Chronic Fatigue Syndrome**
- **Chronic Fatigue and Immune Dysfunction**
- **Fibromyalgia**
- **Hypothyroidism**
- **Chronic Sinusitis**
- **Atopic Eczema**
- **GERD**
- **GI Dysbiosis**
- **Adrenal Dysfunction**
- **Rosacea**

- **Psoriasis**
- **Macular Degeneration**
- **Barrett's Esophagus**
- **Lactose Intolerance**
- **Gluten and Casein Intolerance**
- **Meniere's Disease**
- **Lupus**
- **Obsessive Compulsive Disorder**
- crawling skin, rashes, itching
- dry and flaking skin
- eczema
- dermatitis
- acne, rosacea
- skin discoloration, blotchiness
- dandruff
- chronic athlete's foot
- chronic toenail/fingernail fungus
- depression
- irritability

- anxiety
- panic attacks
- recurring obsessive thoughts
- personality changes, mood swings
- paranoia
- joints pain, muscle aches
- tightness shoulders, neck
- brown colored mucus
- sore throat
- low-grade fever, low body temp
- projectile vomiting

Common Symptoms of Candida Overgrowth

Metabolic/Digestion Symptoms	Mental/Emotional Symptoms	Whole Body Symptoms
Weight gain, obesity	Headaches, migraines	Chronic fatigue
Increased belly fat	Sleep problems	Muscle weakness
High carbs, sugar, alcohol cravings	Night sweats	Irregular heartbeat
Cravings for dairy, sour foods	Lack of concentration	Cold hands & feet
Bulimia or anorexia	Mood swings	Allergies, acne, eczema, dandruff
Indigestion, acid reflux	Increased irritability	Frequent infections
Bloating, gas	High anxiety	Asthma / persistent cough
IBS (irritable bowel syndrome)	Hyperactivity / ADD	Itching, running nose / sinus inflammation
Hypoglycemia	Memory problems	Ear pain / itching
Metabolic syndrome	Brain fog, confusion	Chronic joint pain
Thyroid dysfunction	Indecisiveness	Low sex drive / impotence
Oral thrush	Sense of floating	Painful intercourse
Constipation/diarrhea	Learning disabilities	Fungal infections
PMS (pre-menstrual syndrome)	Depression	Rectal / vaginal itching

BrainyWeightLoss.com

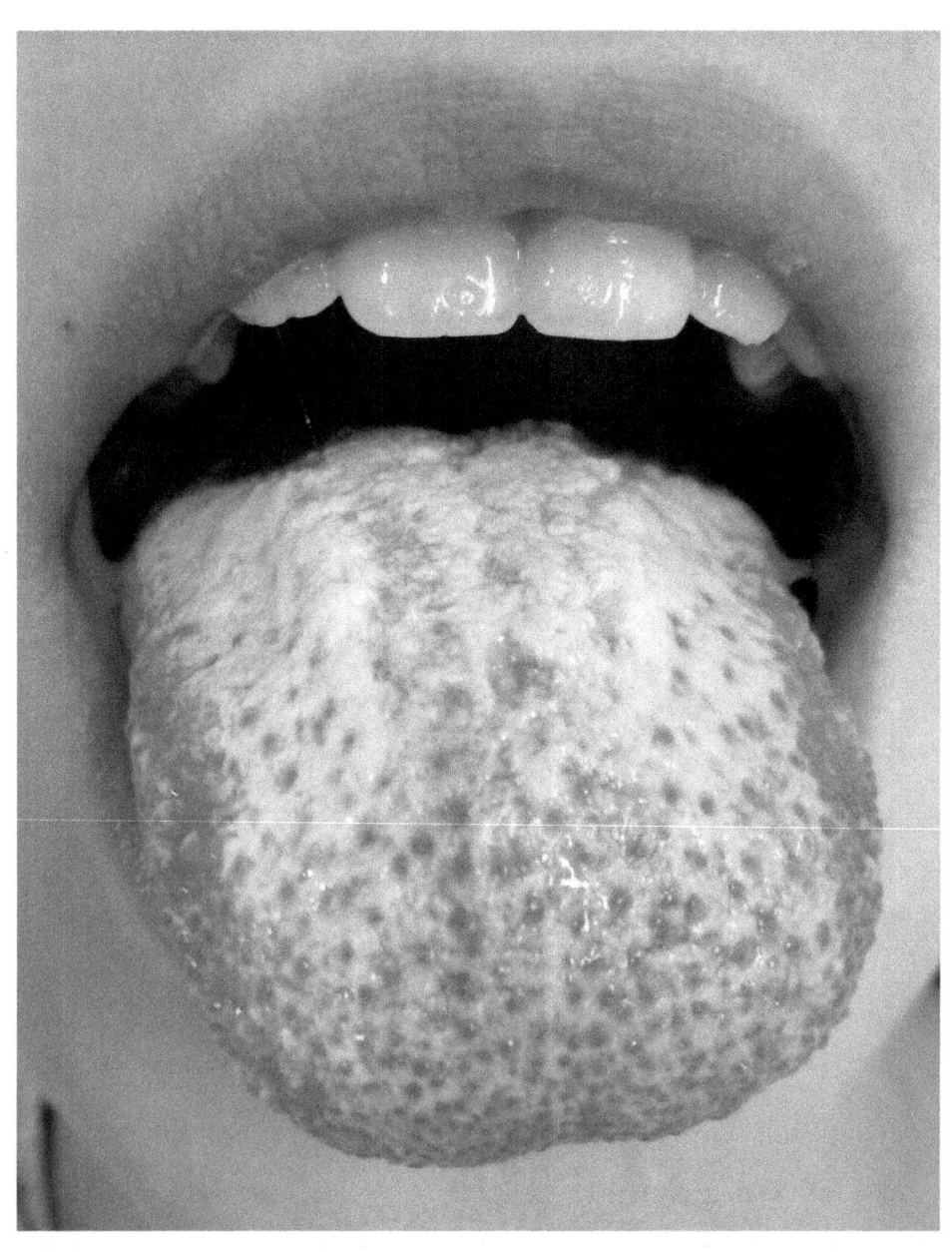

Tongue coated with Candida

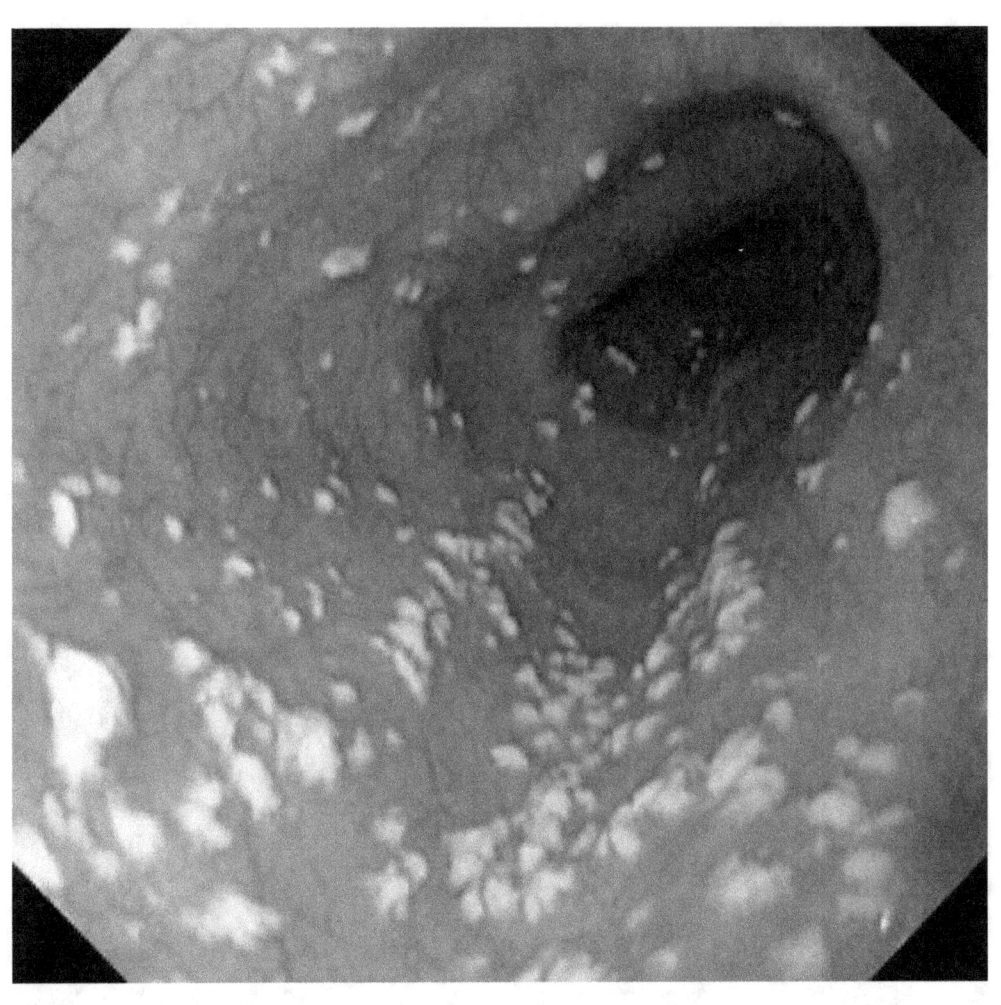

Colon infected with candida overgrowth

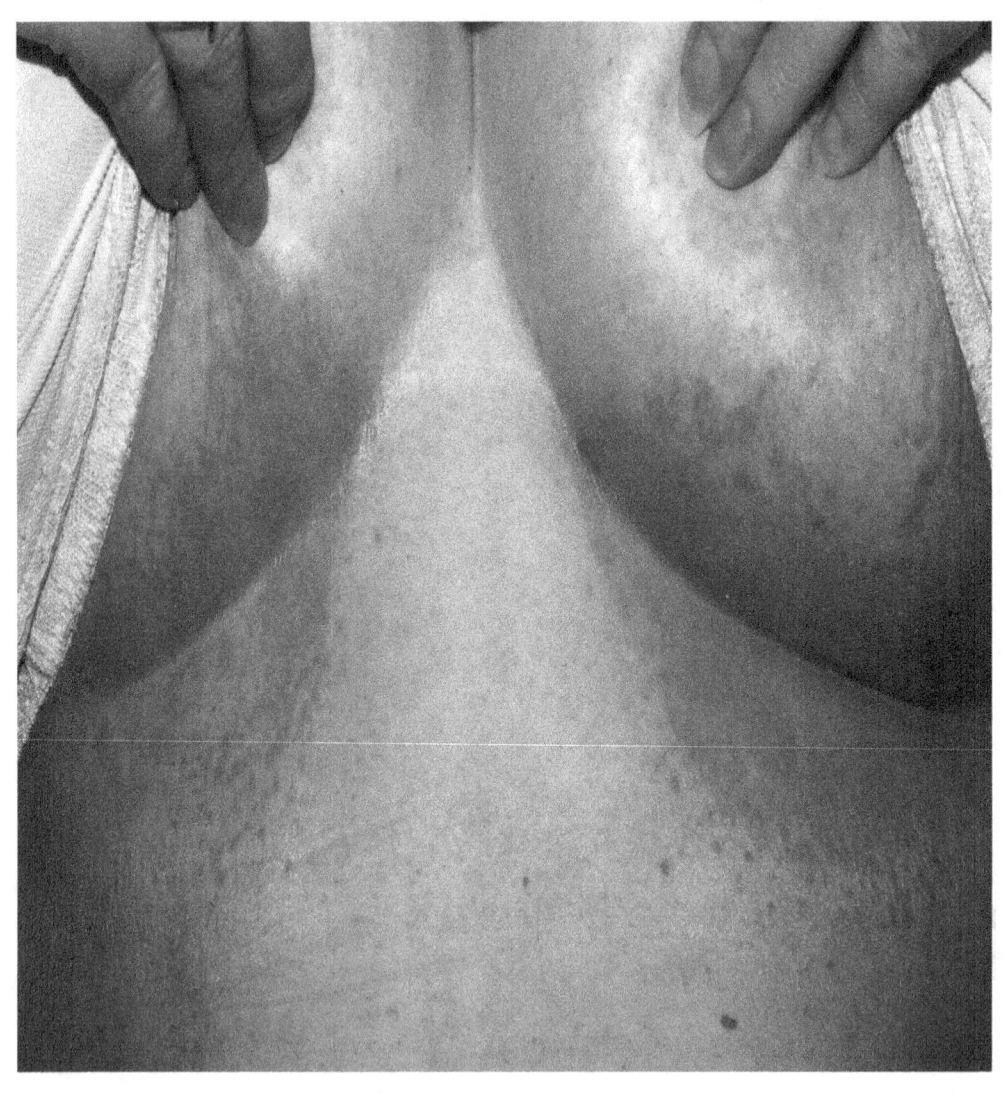

Candida rash under breasts

2.4 Current methods of diagnosis

There are fortunately a variety of methods for aiding in diagnosing candida. I will go over a number of them, some a bit controversial and others requiring blood and stool work.

CULTURE:

As per the CDC: Healthcare providers rely on your medical history, symptoms, physical examinations, and laboratory tests to diagnose invasive candidiasis. The most common way that healthcare providers test for invasive candidiasis is by taking a blood sample or sample from the infected body site and sending it to a laboratory to see if it will grow *Candida* in a culture. A culture can be done with saliva, stool or with blood. It is relatively accurate but requires a healthcare provider such as a doctor to run the test.

BLOOD TEST:

Another test utilizing blood is the Candida antibody IgA lab. While this also usually requires a doctor's prescription things have happily changed in this area. You can now get many labs done without a doctor by making use of the many online labs. In this case, you as the consumer can purchase a lab and the company's doctor will sign the order for you and send you with an order to such labs as LABCORP or Quest. One of the best out here along with discounted rates for the labs is Walk-In-Lab at **www.walkinlab.com.** The lab you would request is called the Candida Antibodies Blood Test, IgA, ELISA test #163020.

AT HOME SPIT TEST.

This is a bit more controversial. I have had many patients do this test instead of spending money for a more thorough test. It can be accurate but it really depends on what you ate just before it and I have seen false negatives many times.

It is done in the morning with the day's first saliva. When you awake in the morning, before you put anything into your mouth, work up some saliva and spit it into a clear glass of water. Within 1-3 minutes, look in the glass. If there are strings coming down from your saliva, or if the water turned cloudy, or if your saliva sank to the bottom, you most likely have candida. Healthy saliva will simply float on the top.

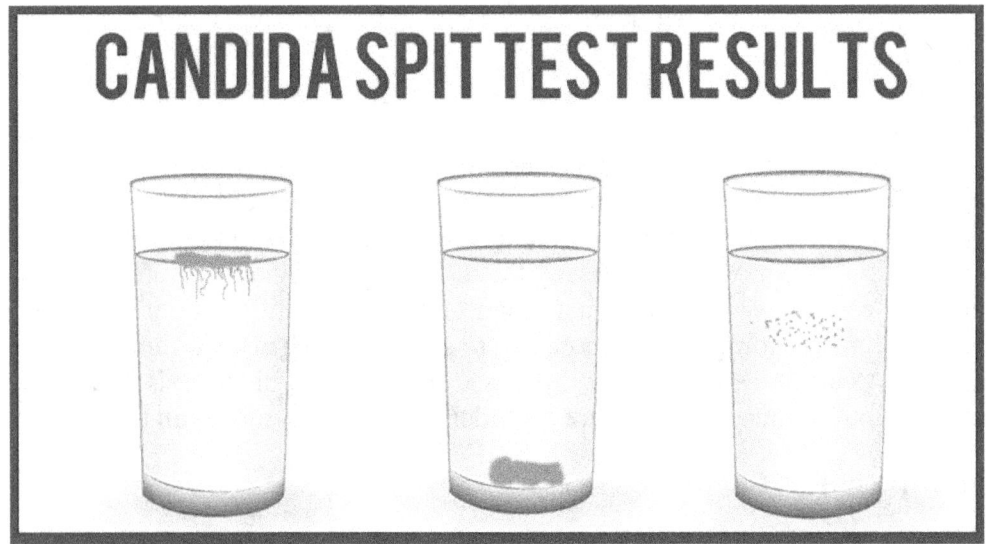

2.5 Conventional methods of treatment

Today we are now aware that in many cases it is antibiotics which can initiate a yeast overgrowth, and, even when they are simply used to treat the condition, they can actually make the problem worse. Some doctors today will still order antibiotics for this condition, seemingly unaware it will simply return, worse than before.

Most will go to the pharmacy and pick up an over-the-counter anti-fungal cream, usually in the case of vaginal infections. At first, it appears to alleviate the problem but in short order it will return as the root cause was not addressed. In this case it means the candida that is rampant on the inside of the body was not treated. In the end, the candida will eventually come back out again.

Most of the time the following anti-fungals are often recommended, with limited success:

- Butoconozole
- Clotrimazole
- Miconazole
- Terconazole

- Clotrimazole (Lotrimin, Mycelex)
- Fluconazole (Diflucan)
- Miconazole (Monistat, Micatin)
- Terconazole (Terazol)

Again, all of the above treatments only temporarily alleviate the symptoms. It WILL come back until you eliminate it from the inside out.

- Drugs, creams and lotions are designed to tackle the symptoms of yeast infections, not its root cause. This is why most conventional treatments for candida infection which work as a temporary band aid solution, fail to work in the long run.

- Even probiotic therapy which is considered as an alternative natural treatment that re-establishes the balance between the good bacteria and the bad bacteria in your digestive tract, fails to work in the long run simply because the root cause of Candida infection is still ignored

Conventional methods do not work in the long run

2.6 Holistic Treatment – The Candida Cleanse.

The first step in my program is to aid the patient in returning the immune system back to a state where it can begin to fight the disease. Since one of the most common disorders affecting the immune system in this country is a candida overgrowth, we start with a cleanse to purge the body of excess of candida and begin to re-establish the micro-flora environment.

One of the main mistakes made with most candida programs is that they will either do a medication protocol or a dietary one but not both. Ours includes both. This is done in a 4 step process combined with a specific dietary plan. You will see below procedures one through four describing the holistic medications taken and the dosages within each step. A medication chart is included in this chapter. The dietary menu plan included in this chapter is done at the same time as steps one through three, starting with day one of step one.

First procedure: Take five capsules five times a day of Dr. Christopher's Intestinal Sweep Formula. This procedure will kill off the yeast, which on other programs can make you feel very nauseous. This nauseous feeling is avoided by taking plant-based digestive enzymes in large amounts (triple the stated dosages on the label) and flushing out with Dr. Christopher's Lower Bowel formula during these first two days. NOTES: The Lower Bowel formula can be taken the whole time if needed. It is best to have 3 bowels movements a day and the amount of Lower Bowel taken is the amount needed to give you 3 bowel movements a day. It is most important during that first procedure so that the body is eliminating the yeast etc. Udo's Choice or Garden of Life have plant-based digestive enzymes, which are available at most herb shops.

Second procedure: For the next 14 days, take five capsules five times per day of Dr. Christopher's Soothing Digestion formula, or one tablespoon of slippery elm gruel five times a day. Either of these methods will coat, soothe and heal the lesions in the intestinal wall. (You can continue to take the

Intestinal Sweep Formula 2 capsules 3 times a day during this time as well as the Lower Bowel.)

Third procedure: For the next two days repeat the first procedure.

Fourth procedure: Take copious (triple the stated dosages on the label) amounts of multi-strain Probiotics to re-establish the flora. Further aids would be to eat raw sauerkraut, Kim Chi, raw apple cider vinegar, Rejuvelac, or miso in large amounts, which are the exact foods to stay away from if you have leaky gut syndrome, yet they rebuild the flora once the leaky gut is healed. NOTES: Udo's Choice has Probiotics, are available at most herb shops. Make sure you look for probiotics with the most strains, not how many billions there are of them. The probiotics need to be taken for about a week to rebuild the flora. Note: It is absolutely essential that you do not feed the yeast during this procedure. Therefore, do not consume any sugar or alcohol in any form. This includes all dairy, grains, and fruit. This is twenty days of a wonderful vegetable, nuts, seeds and sprouted legume diet; thus insuring a healthy life, free of Systemic Yeast Overgrowth. This step is meant to regrow your "garden". Please, during these two months eat as many of the above fermented foods as well as probiotics because not one food or product carries all of the 1400 different strains you need. You do not want a "mono-crop" but a very diverse and healthy "garden" or immune system **since 70% to 80% of your immune system resides in your gut.**

Please note how to read the included medication chart. The codes for the medications are as follows:

IS – Intestinal Sweep.
LB – Lower Bowel.
SD = Soothing Digestion.

So, far example, on day one of step one at 7:00 in the morning it shows 5-IS/2-LB. This means to take 5 Intestinal Sweep and 2 Lower Bowels. Be aware of how the dosages change for each hour and each step in the program.

It is important to know that this cleanse can cause a very significant detox or what is called a Herx response. During a candida die-off, mycotoxins are released and they can make you feel pretty sick. You may experience headaches, gas, bloating, muscle and joint pain, depression, anxiety and even flu-like symptoms. Not everyone experiences them but the worse your candida overgrowth is, the stronger the symptoms may be. The worst of the die-off is usually in step one since this will be the time of the greatest amount of dying candida due to the Intestinal Sweep medication.

There are a couple of "tricks" you can do to help make it through the detox. The first is very simple, drink LOTS of water. The more you drink, the faster the blood is flushed and the less side-effects you may experience. So, if you are feeling pretty bad, it is a clear sign to drink MORE water.

The second "trick" is a bit more complex. It requires a licensed hydro-therapist and utilizes a protocol called a colonic. This is not required and most patients have not needed to take advantage of it. But, for those feeling the effects strongly, a colonic can be very helpful done on day three, when the majority of the die-off has already occurred. Right after the colonic you may notice a significant improvement in your overall well being.

Please make a special note of how the medications and their dosages change in each step. The included medication sheet can become your friend if you pay attention to the schedule. Many patients end up putting it on the refrigerator and mark off each dosage as they take their medications.

Once you get to day 19, you are now done with the candida medication portion of the program and it will be time to take plenty of the probiotics and fermented foods. Many patients ask at this time if they can go back to their old diets. Obviously, the answer is no. That is part of what got you where you are at. It recommended that for at least the first two weeks of step four to remain on the candida diet to allow the micro-flora to begin to populate. At the start of step four you are basically working with a blank slate and you will need to give it some time to colonize enough bacteria to hold the candida in check. This means there is no sugar, not even from fruit. Otherwise you are very likely to have the candida over grow again.

After two weeks you can begin to SLOWLY reintroduce fruits back into your diet. I still recommend a healthy, vegan diet for the rest of your life if you are looking for a more permanent and complete healing of your body.

CANDIDA MENU PLAN

As stated earlier, the following menu plan is to be started on day one of step and to continue though all of the first three steps. This is a vegan, sugar and alcohol free diet meant to starve the candida while the medications kill the yeast. Any vegetable is allowed except for very starchy types such as potatoes. Carrots in moderation.

Monday

Breakfast: Oatmeal(using the thermos method) with almond milk(unsweetened) add tsp of cinnamon Sprinkle on some hulled hemp seeds.

Midmorning: juice with celery, parsley, and spinach

Lunch: salad with mixed greens, cucumber with garlic, lemon, olive and flax oil dressing. 1 carrot and 1celery stick. Hand full of walnuts.

Dinner: Tempeh or Tofu (organic or GMO free) stir fry with brown rice and tahini sauce, grilled/baked vegetables (zucchini, onion, garlic, and squash) green salad with a garlic, lemon and olive oil dressing.

Tuesday

Breakfast: Oatmeal(using the thermos method) with almond milk(unsweetened) add tsp of cinnamon

Midmorning: juice with cucumber, 1 carrot, parsley

Lunch: Green salad or bean salad (no sugar), avocado, green onion with garlic and oil, grilled vegetables

Dinner: Vegan Sushi rolls(use brown rice only) made with avocado, carrot and mushroom. Green salad made with Tahini dressing and sunflower seeds)

Wednesday

Breakfast: Oatmeal(using the thermos method) with almond milk(unsweetened) add tsp of cinnamon

Midmorning: juice with celery, parsley, and mixed greens

Lunch: Green salad with spinach, sunflower seeds, cucumber, with garlic, lemon, ginger and olive oil dressing.

Dinner: vegan pattie on 2 slices of Ezekiel bread or **Vegetable Quinoa**, Add slice of tomato, Mushrooms, onion with 2 carrot and celery sticks. Green salad with tahini dressing.

Thursday

Breakfast: Oatmeal(using the thermos method) with almond milk(unsweetened) add tsp of cinnamon.

Midmorning: juice with cucumber, parsley, and spinach

Lunch: Green salad with cabbage, green onion, 1/2 grated carrot, with ginger, oil, lemon, garlic, and dill for dressing, hand full of walnuts.

Dinner: grilled or steamed vegetables over brown rice. Sliced tomato 1 slice of Ezekiel bread. Hummus with radishes or celery.

Friday

Breakfast: Oatmeal(using the thermos method) with almond milk(unsweetened) add tsp of cinnamon.

Midmorning: juice with celery, parsley.

Lunch: salad with Romaine Lettuce, avocado, green onion with Garlic and oil dressing, black bean soup with grilled vegetables

Dinner: vegan burger (see above on what to add) or **Vegetable Quinoa** with a green salad or Sushi rolls.

Saturday

Breakfast: Oatmeal(using the thermos method) with almond milk(unsweetened) add tsp of cinnamon

Midmorning: juice with celery, parsley, and mixed greens

Lunch: Green salad with spinach, sunflower seeds, cucumber, with garlic, lemon, ginger and olive oil dressing.

Dinner: vegan pattie on 2 slices of Ezekiel bread or **Vegetable Quinoa**, Add slice of tomato, Mushrooms, onion with 2 carrot and celery sticks. Green salad with tahini dressing.

Sunday

Breakfast: Oatmeal(using the thermos method) with almond milk(unsweetened) add tsp of cinnamon

Midmorning: juice with cucumber, 1 carrot, parsley

Lunch: Green salad or bean salad (no sugar), avocado, green onion with garlic and oil, grilled vegetables

Dinner: Vegan Sushi rolls(use brown rice only) made with avocado, carrot and mushroom. Green salad made with Tahini dressing and sunflower seeds)

You can also snack on black bean soup, parsley soup, and vegetable broth in rotation. It is fine to mix and match.

If you like you can add PLAIN(NO SUGAR) plant-based yogurt to any of the days. Maybe have a cup for breakfast instead of Oatmeal or add it with the oatmeal.

**For your plant-based yogurt you can add a few walnuts or sunflower seeds.

**Hummus can be used on the vegan burgers or use as a dressing.

The above menu plan is very simple. The general rule of thumb is: if the food is one the menu plan you can eat it, if not, than you should not. All vegetables are included except for potatoes and other very starchy types.

CANDIDA SNACKS

Popcorn

As a general rule, increasing your fiber intake can help control candida. Air-popped popcorn is a high-fiber snack recommended by Free-fad-diets.com. Make your own popcorn and add a little vegan butter and salt if desired. Avoid pre-popped popcorn snacks that may contain sugars or yeast-based flavorings.

Nuts and Seeds

Free-fad-diets.com recommends sunflower and pumpkin seeds, nuts and almond or cashew butters for snacking on a candida diet. Spread nut butters on yeast-free and white-flour-free crackers, rice crisps or oat crisps.

If plain almonds grew a little tiresome, I'd try something a little more elaborate: spice-toasted almonds.

- 1/2 tsp turmeric
- 1/2 tsp xylitol
- 1/4 tsp ground ginger
- Pinch cumin
- Pinch cayenne pepper
- 1/4 tsp sea salt
- 1/2 cup freshly shelled almonds

Put the first six ingredients in a bowl and mix. Toss your almonds in the Braggs liquid aminos, then in your spice mixture. Toast under your grill, turning once they've browned on one side or, if your oven's on for something else, bake in the oven at about 375° for about 12-14 minutes until dry.

Vegetables with Dips

We recommend pureeing chickpeas with some tahini for a hummus dip to eat with vegetable sticks or slices. White cannellini beans pureed with garlic and enough olive oil for the desired consistency is another dip option. Add mint, chives or thyme to boost the flavor.

Guacamole

Combine fresh avocados, onions and tomatoes to make your own guacamole dip. Use organic, sugar-free corn tortillas, or buy organic, sugar-free corn chips.

Coconut

We suggest fresh coconut as a snack. Crack open a coconut and keep it in the refrigerator, ready for snacking. Avoid packaged or frozen coconut, which typically has sugar added.

Chickpeas

Chickpeas, the main ingredient in hummus, are also a good snack right from the can. Season them lightly with salt and pepper, if desired. Add some ground coriander seeds, or add minced garlic or garlic powder for extra flavor.

Snack Ideas

Take a look at the following food list for the Candida diet that can be consumed as snacks, along with some suggestions on combining them together for a delicious and filling snack.

Almond or Cashew Butter Spreads (Avoid Peanut Butter)
Vegetables
Garlic Products
Coconut
Tahini
Humus
Air-Popped Popcorn (not the commercial variety)
Soy/coconut/almond Yogurt (plain)
Nuts and Seeds such as Almonds, Pecans, Macadamia (Peanuts and Pistachios not allowed), Pumpkin seeds, Sunflower Seeds, Sesame Seeds (unsalted)
Unsweetened carob chips
(Brown) Rice Crackers
Soy Milk/Rice Milk (unsweetened)

Homemade Tortilla Chips or Yeast-Free Commercial Varieties
Homemade Salsa
Sprouted Grain Bread

SOME RECIPES:

ALMOND MILK – No sugar

As for almond milk being expensive to make, here is how I do it very cheaply:
1 cup raw almond soaked for 4 hours or more (I do overnight).
4 cups filtered or distilled water.

Pinch of salt

A few drops of vanilla (optional)

In a high speed blender or a vita mix blend nuts and water for about two minutes.
Then filter through a double cheesecloth or cotton diaper the milk and save it and compost the leftover meat.

Put milk back into blender and add the other ingredients and blend again. AWESOME!

Refrigerate and that's it.
Very cheap and easy and raw. That is what I do.

The name of the coffee substitute is Roma.

OATMEAL THERMOS METHOD

Instructions for the Oatmeal:

Now... there is a way to get some oats in a safe and very tasty manner. I am going to include a method here for making oatmeal which is still VERY high in enzymes, vitamins, minerals and produces an alkaline reaction. Here you go:

You will need:

1.) Oat Groats. You can get them at the health food store and grain stores. Make SURE they are OAT GROATS and organic if you can, not steel cut, nothing else.

2.) Water, preferred distilled of course.

3.) A good thermos, not steel lined but glass lined interior.

We usually do this about 7:00 or so in the evening prior to the morning that we would like them for breakfast.

OK, pour the oat groats into the thermos until it is 1/4 to 1/3 full of them. Boil the water and then pour into thermos until about an inch of air space is left at the top. This is so the oat groats can expand over night. Close tight the thermos and shake well. Then place on the kitchen counter until morning.

In the morning pop the top and the oats should still be nice and warm and smelling wonderful! Stevia is accepted as a sweetener on this cleanse.

Candida/Leaky Gut Syndrome Cleanse Schedule

IS = Intestinal Sweep   **LB** = Lower Bowel   **SD** = Soothing Digestion

	Date	7:00am	10:00am	1:00pm	4:00pm	7:00pm
Step 1 2 DAYS Intestinal Sweep IS=50 LB=12		5-IS/2-LB	5-IS	5-IS/2-LB	5-IS	5-IS/2-LB
	1					
	2					
		7:00am	10:00am	1:00pm	4:00pm	7:00pm
		5-SD/2-IS/2-LB	5-SD	5-SD/2-IS/2-LB	5-SD	5-SD/2-IS/2-LB
Step 2 14 DAYS Soothing Digestion SD=350 13 DAYS Intestinal Sweep IS= 78 CONTINUE TO TAKE LOWER BOWEL AS IN STEP ONE	3					
	4					
	5					
	6					
	7					
	8					
	9					
	10					
	11					
	12					
	13					
	14					
	15					
	16					
		7:00am	10:00am	1:00pm	4:00pm	7:00pm
Step 3 2 DAYS Intestinal Sweep IS=50 LB=12		5-IS/2-LB	5-IS	5-IS/2-LB	5-IS	5-IS/2-LB
	17					
	18					
	Select Probiotic of Choice					
Step 4 2 MOS Re-establish Flora: *Probiotics 3x label dosage or Large Amounts of: *Raw Sauerkraut *Kim Chi *Raw Apple Cider Vinegar *Rejuvelac *Miso	19					

Herbs required: 2 Bottles-Soothing Digestion   1 Bottle-Intestinal Sweep   1 Bottle-Lower Bowel

Notes: You should have 3 bowel movements a day. This is most important during the first procedure so that the body is eliminating the yeast, etc... If necessary, the Lower Bowel formula can be taken the entire time. In some cases, a colonic might be necessary.

CHAPTER 3

Parasites

3.1 What are parasites and how common are they?

As stated by the CDC, "**A parasite is an organism that lives on or in a host organism and gets its food from or at the expense of its host. There are three main classes of parasites that can cause disease in humans: protozoa, helminths, and ectoparasites.**"

Protozoa are microscopic, one-celled organisms that can be free-living or parasitic in nature. They are able to multiply in humans, which contributes to their survival and also permits serious infections to develop from just a single organism. Transmission of protozoa that live in a human's intestine to another human typically occurs through a fecal-oral route (for example, contaminated food or water or person-to-person contact). Protozoa that live in the blood or tissue of humans are transmitted to other humans by an arthropod vector (for example, through the bite of a mosquito or sand fly).

Helminths are large, multi-cellular organisms that are generally visible to the naked eye in their adult stages. Like protozoa, helminths can be either free-living or parasitic in nature. In their adult form, helminths cannot multiply in humans. There are three main groups of helminths (derived from the Greek word for worms) that are human parasites: Flatworms, Thorny-headed worms and Roundworms.

Ectoparasites can broadly include blood-sucking arthropods such as mosquitoes (because they are dependent on a blood meal from a human host for their survival), this term is generally used more narrowly to refer to organisms such as ticks, fleas, lice, and mites that attach or burrow into the skin and remain there for relatively long periods of time (e.g., weeks to months). Arthropods are important in causing diseases in their own right, but are even more important as vectors, or transmitters, of many different pathogens that in turn cause tremendous morbidity and mortality from the diseases they cause.

Parasitic infections cause a tremendous burden of disease in both the tropics and subtropics as well as in more temperate climates. Of all parasitic diseases, malaria causes the most deaths globally. Malaria kills approximately 660,000 people each year, most of them young children in sub-Saharan Africa.

The Neglected Tropical Diseases (NTDs), which have suffered from a lack of attention by the public health community, include parasitic diseases such as lymphatic filariasis, onchocerciasis, and Guinea worm disease. The NTDs affect more than 1 billion people—one-sixth of the world's population—largely in rural areas of low-income countries. These diseases extract a large toll on endemic populations, including lost ability to attend school or work, retardation of growth in children, impairment of cognitive skills and development in young children, and the serious economic burden placed on entire countries.

However, parasitic infections also affect persons living in developed countries, including the United States.

According to the CDC, approximately 1 out of 6 Americans have parasites, usually intestinal. I tend to believe this is a conservative estimate. Most patients that we have done stool testing on have had intestinal parasites. There are millions of cases reported each year in this country. An infection can lead to serious health problems, including seizures, blindness, pregnancy complications, heart failure and even death.

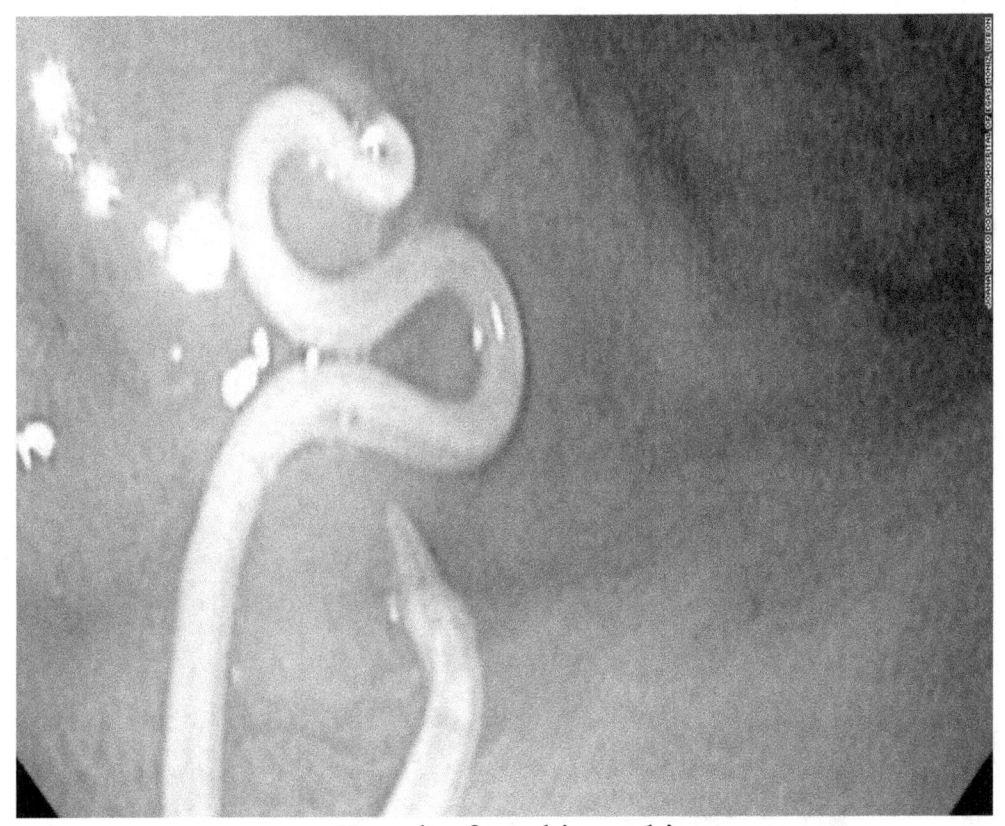

Parasite found in sushi

Web Atlas of Human Parasitology

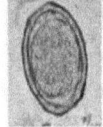 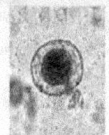 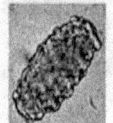 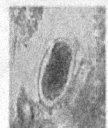 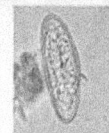 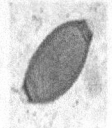 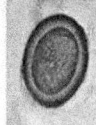 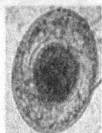

| Ascaris lumbricoides | Ascaris lumbricoides | Ascaris lumbricoides infértil | Ancilostomídeo | Enterobius vermicularis | Trichuris trichiura | Taenia sp. | Hymenolepis sp. |

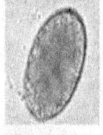 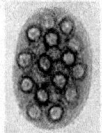 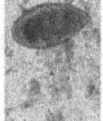 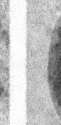 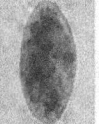 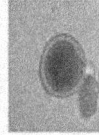 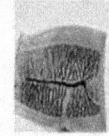 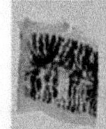 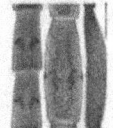

| Diphylobothrium sp. | Dipylidium sp. (aglomerado de ovos) | Schistosoma mansoni | Fasciola hepatica | Toxocara canis | Taenia saginata proglóte | Taenia solium proglóte | Dipylidium sp. proglótes |

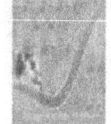 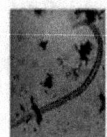 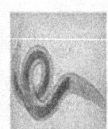 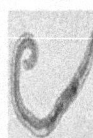 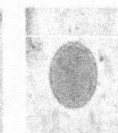 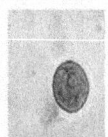 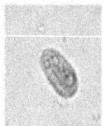 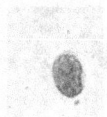

| Strongyloides stercoralis Larva | Ancilostomídeo sp. (larva filarióide) | Enterobius vermicularis (larva femea) | Enterobius vermicularis (larva macho) | Entamoeba coli | Entamoeba histolytica | Giardia lamblia |

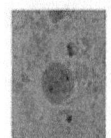 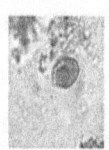 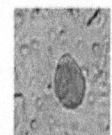 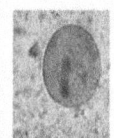 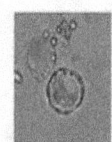 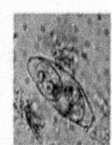 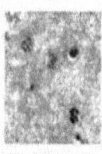 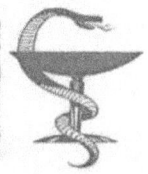

| Endolimax nana | Iodamoeba butschlii | Chilomastix mesnili | Balantidium coli | Blastocystis sp. | Isospora sp. | Cryptosporidium sp. |

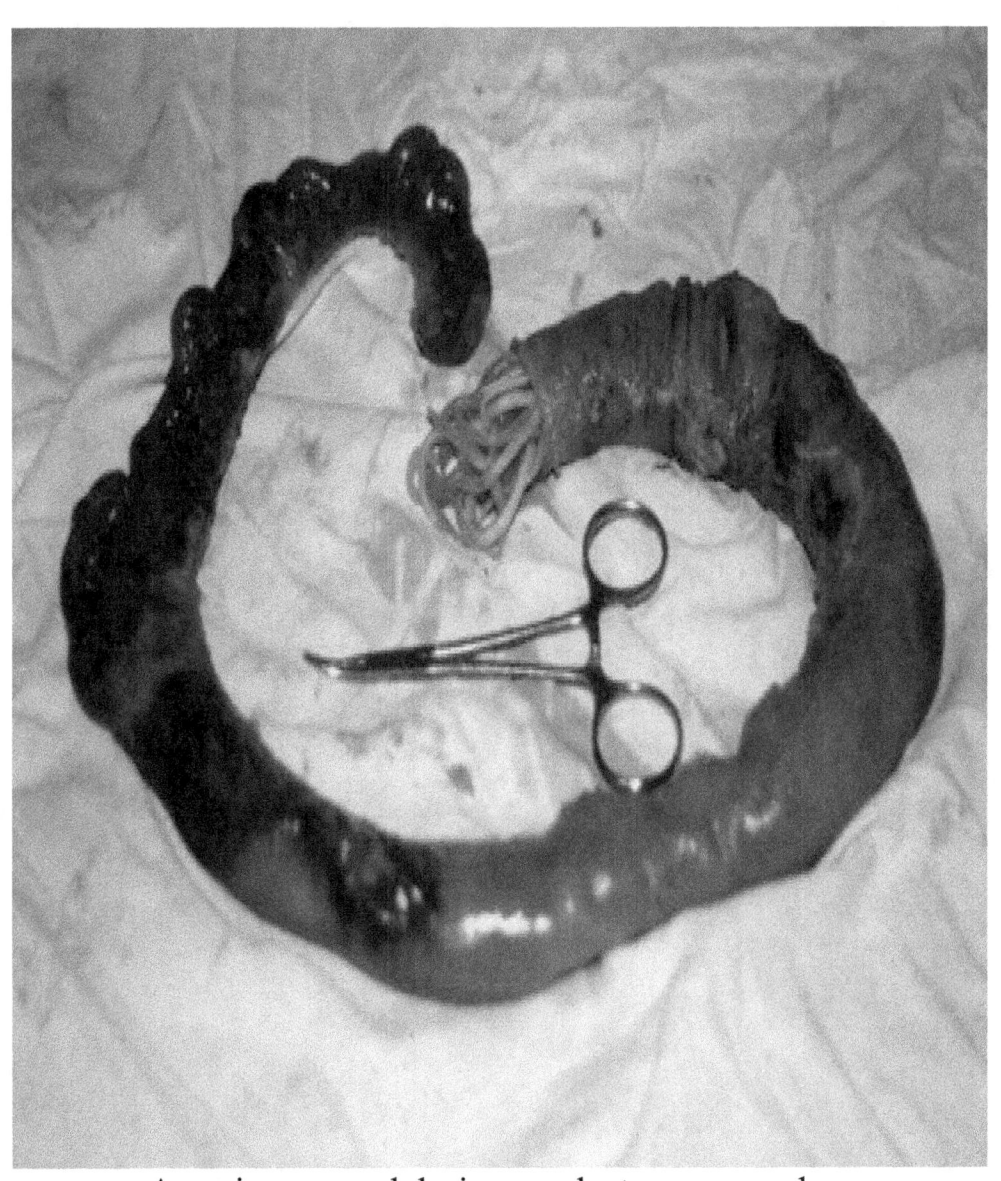
Ascaris removed during a colectomy procedure

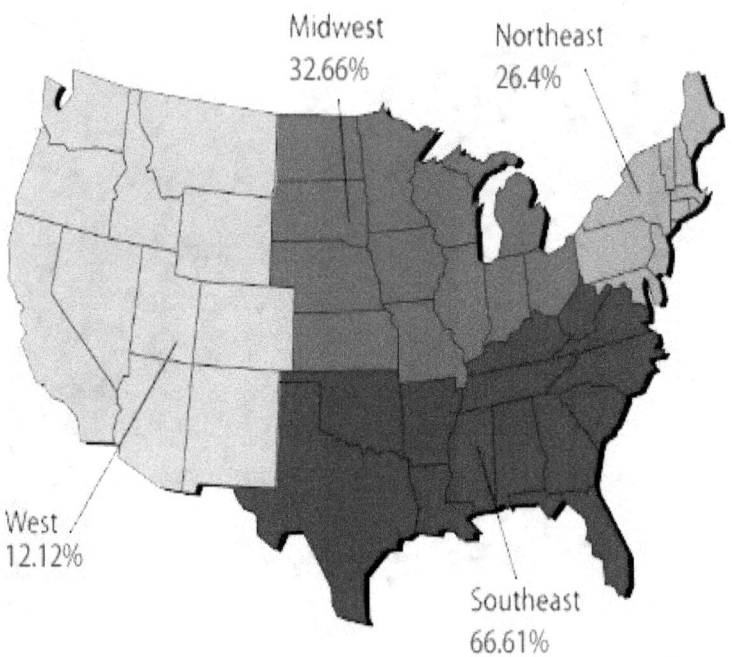

Source: National Prevalence Study Interim Report, Conducted by Dr. Byron Blagburn, MS, PhD, College of Veterinary Medicine, Auburn University, Nov. 2009.

3.2 Causes of Parasites

Parasites enter the body via the mouth, the skin and the bottom of the feet. Direct contact with the bodily fluids of a contaminated person can also spread parasites. Parasites can be found in contaminated soil, vegetables, meat, watercress and feces. Worm eggs or larvae are often ingested in partially or uncooked foods and they can become airborne.

I have seen many cases where the patient would get them from their dogs or cats. If the dog or cats spends a significant amount of time outside and then comes in at night and sleeps in the same bed then transmission can easily occur. Many intestinal parasites come out at night and can move between hosts. It is usually the case when a patient has been diagnosed with parasites we end up treating the whole family; humans, dogs and cats.

Studies show 9 times out of 10 parasite infections are actually lifestyle-induced, not environmentally. That means you are less likely to get a parasite from water than you are from living an unhealthy lifestyle.

The biggest cause of parasite infections is a weakened immune system. It's a two-way street. Living a lifestyle that weakens the immune system is the most likely way to attract a parasitic infection; this is because a weakened body is a breeding ground for them. It is their job as the universal garbage men to clean up waste. A sick body is a wasting body and therefore, food in a parasite's world.

3.3 Symptoms of parasites and related diseases

Symptoms of parasite infestations can be quite varied and mimic a large number of other disorders. Following is a partial list of possible symptoms:

- Strong cravings for processed and sugary foods
- Mood disorders
- Anemia or iron deficiency (worms can create enough blood loss to cause anemia or iron deficiency)
- Skin ailments such as hives, rashes, weeping eczema, itchy dermatitis, acne, ulcers, sores, lesions, etc.
- Recurring yeast infections like Candida
- Bleeding gums
- Headaches
- Anxiety
- Nervousness
- Teeth grinding and drooling during sleep
- Food allergies/food sensitivities
- Loss of appetite
- Sexual dysfunction
- Chronic fatigue

- Unhealthy food cravings

- Persistent digestive problems (cramps, bloating, gas, etc.)

- Hungry all the time

- Sore/stiff joints

- Breathing problems

- Bed wetting (very common with children)

- Itching – especially around mouth, nose and anus

- Memory problems

Look familiar? Yes, they even look very similar to candida symptoms. This is one of the great challenges to discerning the root causes of so many diseases. I usually find it best to treat for both candida and parasites unless I have actual lab evidence of one or the other.

A short list of some of the diseases caused by parasite:

IBS
Autoimmune
Diarrhea
Depression
Anxiety
Sexually transmitted such as Trichomoniasis
Sleeping sickness
Gardiasis
Heartworm disease.
Scabies
Liver diseases
Brain disorders
Chronic vomiting
Chronic fatigue syndrome.

3.4 Current methods of diagnosis

Testing largely depends on the type of parasite. For example, pinworms are the most common parasites residing To test you will have to conduct a tape test for the diagnosis of Pinworm infection. This test is quite simple. All you have to do is to take a piece of cellophane tape and press its sticky side against the skin around the anus. As pinworms usually exit the body during the night, you should do this test in the morning. If they are residing in your body, the eggs will stick to the cellophane tape. Take the tape to your doctor, who will examine it under a slide to check if there are any pinworm eggs on it. Pinworm infection is also called enterobiasis and oxyuriasis. This infection can spread quickly. Adults usually get this infection from pinworm-infected children. This infection does not incur any complications or long-term health effects.

For most other parasites a blood or stool test is usually required. Again, **Walk-In-Lab (walkinlab.com)** has stool kit tests available without the need to go to a local doctor. You can do a search on their site for parasite testing.

Again, this is not meant to be a substitute for going to a qualified health care provider.

3.5 Conventional methods of treatments

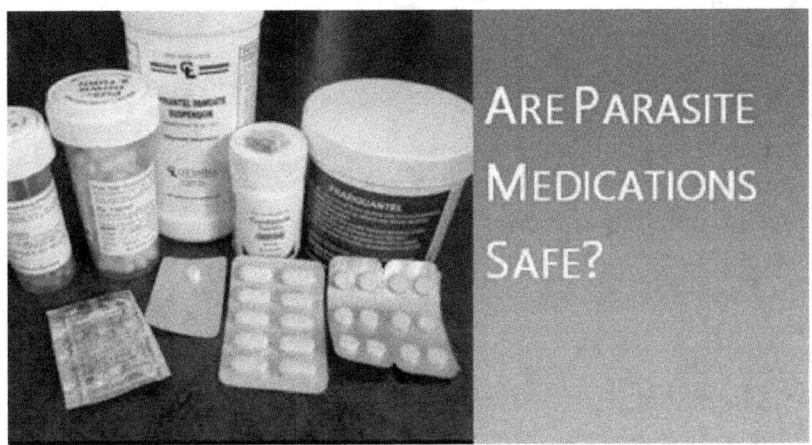

Most types of parasites are treated by medication and thorough cleaning of the house. Moreover, the family members and caregivers of the infected child should also obtain treatment for the Pinworm infection along with implementing a specific hygiene and house-cleaning regimen.

Anti-parasitic drugs, like metronidazole, quinacrine, tinidazole and furazolidone are usually effective, but the exact treatment regime, as prescribed by your doctor, should be followed.

Paramomycin is not absorbed from the intestine into the blood, so it may be used in pregnancy. For cyclospora **trimethoprim-sulfametoxazol** can be used. Intestinal parasites can be successfully eradicated, but may recur if the source of infection still exists. Delayed treatment can lead to a host of complications, some of which can be life threatening, as may be the case of severe dehydration in diseases like giardiasis.

However, you should not take any medication without a doctor's prescription. Be aware that each of the above mentioned drugs can come with significant side effects. Some of the possible side effects include:

- Dizziness
- Diarrhea
- Liver damage
- Fast heartbeat
- Joint or muscle pain
- Red skin lesions
- Hair loss
- Painful or difficult urination
- Upper right abdominal or stomach pain
- Unusual bleeding or bruising
- Sore, ulcers or white spots on the lips or mouth.
- Hives or welts
- Fever
- Convulsions
- Dark urine
- Light colored stools (sign of liver damage)
- Fatigue

Needless to say, the list goes on and on ....

3.6 Holistic treatment – The Parasite Cleanse

As you can see from the above section, while pharmaceuticals may be effective (but not always) they do carry the possibility of a very expensive price tag in regards to your health. This is often the case of the cure being more harmful than the disease.

Fortunately, you have a wide assortment of herbal and holistic medications at your disposal. In this section I will list many of the tried and true remedies that have been used throughout history successfully. Again, please keep in mind this is not intended for you to forego the care of a qualified health care professional.

The good news is that for the most part, the same treatments will work on most intestinal parasites.

A good parasite cleanse should include the following aspects:

- A method for softening/removing old fecal solids from the intestinal tract.
- Holistic medications to kill the parasite and their eggs.
- A diet rich in anti-parasite foods such as garlic, cayenne, etc.
- Probiotics to aid in healing the intestinal tract from the damage the parasites caused.

A large number of herbs are very good at killing the parasites and aiding the body in eliminating them. One of Dr. Christopher's favorites was Pumpkin seeds. As he stated in his literature:

*"**Pumpkin Seeds:** A simple herbal aid for a mild case of worms is to use pumpkin seeds (Cucurbitaceae). It is best when fresh seeds are used. To make the infusion, steep one ounce of crushed seeds for fifteen to twenty minutes in a pint of boiling hot water. Dosage: One teacupful or more (up*

to one pint daily), six days a week for one to three weeks. Also eat one to two ounces of the pumpkin seeds each day.

Another "Seed" Aid is to Combine the Following:
1 part pumpkin seeds, crushed (Cucurbitaceae) 1 part watermelon seeds, crushed (Citrullus vulgaris) 1 part cucumber seeds, crushed (Cucumis sativus)
Dosage: Take one pint of emulsion (two ounces of seeds triturated in honey and distilled water) in doses at two hour intervals; or take one to two tablespoons of the crushed seeds in honey, syrup, etc., in three doses at two hour intervals.

The patient should fast during this treatment, then take an appropriate cathartic several hours after the last dosage such as senna tea or preferably the lower bowel formula. Use this procedure at least three days in a row."

At the clinic we use the following two herbal medications:

- Dr. Christopher's Lower Bowel (or Kid-e-Reg for children)
- Dr. Christopher's VF Syrup

The purpose of the Lower Bowel or Kid-e-Reg is meant to keep the bowels moving to aid in eliminating the dead parasites from the body. As stated by Dr. Christopher *"In most cases, improper diet has caused the peristaltic muscles of most people to quit working, and it will take six to nine months with the aid of the lower bowel tonics for the average individual to clean out the fecal matter and to rebuild the bowel structure sufficiently to have the peristaltic muscles work entirely on their own. Most people have pounds of old dried fecal matter that is stored in the colon which is toxifying the system and keeping the food from being assimilated."*

The ingredients are as follows:

1 part Barberry bark (Berberis vulgaris)
2 parts Cascara sagrada bark (Rhamnus purshiana)
1 part Cayenne (Capsicum minimum)
1 part Ginger (Zingiber officinale)

1 part Golden seal root (Hydrastis canadensis)
1 part Lobelia herb and/or seeds (Lobelia inflata)
1 part Red raspberry leaves (Rubus idaeus)
1 part Turkey rhubarb root (Rheum palmatum)
1 part Fennel (Foeniculum vulgari)

The recommended dosage for adults is two capsules three times a day throughout the full treatment.

The VF formula is used to kill the parasites. Again, as stated by Dr. Christopher *"This combination is to act as a vermifuge (a combination that will cause expulsion of worms from the body) and/or a vermicide (herbal agent that destroys worms in the body). "*

The ingredients are as follows:

Wormwood
American wormseed
Tame sage
Fennel
Male fern
Papaya

The recommended dosage for adults is to take one teaspoon each morning and night for three days. On the fourth day drink one cup of senna and peppermint tea (1/2 and 1/2). Rest two days and repeat two more times.

There are also a number of single herbs which have been used historically for removing parasites:

- **Walnut**: This is one of my favorites. More recently some have found the walnut to be effective against intestinal parasites by taking two to three ounces of walnut oil each evening for three days.
- **Hazelnut**: The ancients considered the hazelnut to be the most wholesome and nourishing of any other shell fruit. The hazelnut is the best digested of all oil-bearing fruits. It is used to destroy intestinal parasites by taking one tablespoonful of the oil in the morning for two weeks.

- **Garlic**: Give 10-30 drops of the fresh juice or 1 teaspoon of garlic syrup.
- **Wormwood**: Round worms (vermifuge). Take 2 fluid ounces to 1 teacup of the infusion night and morning, or take the dosage night and morning and an active cathartic every 2nd or 3rd morning; or take 10 - 30 grains of powder night and morning, followed by an appropriate cathartic as indicated;... This will clean the worms from the stomach and leave it toned up.

As always in any proper holistic protocol, **diet** is one of the most important, if not the most important aspect of the program. A clean, vegan diet has been found to be incredibly effective in starving the parasites while using holistic medications to kill and eliminate them.

CHAPTER 4

Heavy Metal Toxicity

4.1 What are heavy metals

HEAVY METAL TOXICITY IS THE ACCUMULATION OF HEAVY METALS, IN TOXIC AMOUNTS, IN THE SOFT TISSUES.

As defined by the NCBI, heavy metals are defined as metallic elements that have a relatively high density compared to water. With the assumption that heaviness and toxicity are inter-related, heavy metals also include metalloids, such as arsenic, that are able to induce toxicity at low level of exposure. In recent years, there has been an increasing ecological and global public health concern associated with environmental contamination by these metals. Also, human exposure has risen dramatically as a result of an exponential increase of their use in several industrial, agricultural, domestic and technological applications. Reported sources of heavy metals in the environment include geogenic, industrial, agricultural, pharmaceutical, domestic effluents, and atmospheric sources. Environmental pollution is very prominent in point source areas such as mining, foundries and smelters, and other metal-based industrial operations. Heavy metal poisoning is caused by the accumulation of certain metals in the body due to exposure through food, water, industrial chemicals, or other sources.

So, all said and done, just what does that mean? It means that some metals and chemicals are becoming more common in this world and we are being exposed to them at an alarming rate and our health is paying the cost. Metals such arsenic, mercury, cadmium, copper, lead, etc. are being absorbed into our bodies and damaging our immune system, much like parasites and candida. See a pattern growing here?

Toxic Elements & Heavy Metals
What limits have been established so far?

	EPA	FDA	USP	WHO/FAO		EU	EU	CA PROP 65
	Drinking Water		Oral Limit	Food	Water	EU Directive 1881/2006	EFSA/ CONTAM Panel	
	mg/L (unless specified)		ppm			mg/kg wet weight	Total Weekly Intake (TWI)	
Aluminum	50-200 µg/L	—	5,000	—	100-200 µg/L	—	—	—
Arsenic (inorganic)	0.01	Apple Juice: 10 ppb	1.5	Provisional Tolerable Weekly Intake (PTWI) 15 µg/kg body weight	10 µg/L	—	No limit; panel says it needs more data.	10 mcg daily intake
Cadmium	0.005	Food Color Additives: 15 ppm	2.5	Provisional Tolerable Monthly Intake (PTMI) 25 µg/kg body weight	3 µg/L	.05 – 3.0	2.5 µg/kg per bw	4.1 mcg daily intake
Copper	1.3	—	50	—	2,000 µg/L	—	—	—
Lead	0.015	Total Daily Intake (TDI) 75 mcg/day Bottled Water: 5 µg/L Candy: 0.1 ppm Fruit Juices: 50 ppb	1	Previous limit withdrawn in 2011.	10 µg/L	.02 – 3.0	Previous limit withdrawn in 2013.	0.5 mcg daily intake
Mercury	0.002	Elemental: 1 ppm	1.5	PTWI 1.6 µg/kg per bw	Inorganic: 6 µg/L	0.1 – 1.0	Inorganic Mercury: 4 µg/kg bw Methylmercury: 1.3 µg/kg bw	0.3 mcg daily intake
Tin	—	—	3,000	PTWI 14 mg/kg per bw	—	50 – 200	—	—

4.2 Causes of heavy metal toxicity

Heavy metal toxicity is now so prevalent that even babies are being born with this condition. A 2004 study by the Environmental Working Group (EWG) found that blood samples from newborns contained an average of 287 toxins, including mercury, fire retardants, pesticides and chemicals in non-stick cookware.

According to the website **www.Theheartysoul.com,** heavy metal toxicity can result from either acute or chronic exposure to heavy metals. Chronic exposure commonly comes from mercury-based amalgam fillings, chemical residues in foods, mercury in vaccines and flu shots, toxins in personal care products, household products, industrial exposures, air and water pollution to name a few. Some professions carry a higher risk for heavy metal exposure such as anyone in the dental profession (including dental office staff), hairdressers, artists, and lab workers.

Individuals who have chronic conditions or weakened immune systems can be more susceptible in developing heavy metal toxicity, as they are not able to excrete these toxins as efficiently as someone with a stronger disposition. Many times, symptoms of metal toxicity are misdiagnosed as chronic illnesses such as multiple sclerosis, chronic fatigue, autism or depression.

Causes of Heavy Metal Poisoning include the following (not a complete list)

- Industrial exposure
- Air or water pollution
- Foods
- Medicines

- Improperly coated food containers, plates, and cookware
- Ingestion of lead-based paints
- Mishandled metals at job site
- Chemical and heavy metal spills
- Living in a home built prior to 1978 that has lead-based paint
- Living near a landfill
- Smoking and/or inhaling second hand smoke
- Eating fish.
- Mercury amalgam fillings

Heavy Metals poisoning

- The most common cause of heavy metal poisoning is lead. Lead poisoning is most common in affluent countries, due to removal of lead from paint, petrol and food cans.

- Mercury can be found in the elemental state (dental amalgam, thermometers), inorganic (industrial processes) and organic compounds (pesticides, wood preservatives, some medicines, and contaminated fish). Ingestion of disc batteries by children can also lead to heavy metal poisoning amongst other problems.

- Poisoning from other heavy metals most often occurs in individuals regularly exposed to the metals in their work environment.

4.3 Symptoms of heavy metal toxicity and related diseases

As you will notice, the symptoms of heavy metal toxicity can be strangely familiar to candida and parasites. One of the main reasons for this is that all three of these conditions adversely affect the immune system, suppressing it and allowing our bodies to be open to opportunistic infections and other disorders.

As with the other conditions, the symptoms may be in the acute or chronic areas. Some of the acute symptoms are as follows:

- Panic
- Headaches
- Convulsions
- Nausea
- Pain
- Vomiting
- Cramping
- Sweating
- Difficulty breathing and other bronchial types conditions
- Impaired cognitive functions

The chronic or long term symptoms may appear after many months or even years:

- Chronic fatigue syndrome
- Chronic infections (due to suppressed immune system)
- General malaise
- Nervous system malfunction manifested as burning, tingling, paralysis,
- Weakness
- Candida (Who knew?)
- Migraines or headaches
- Insomnia

- Brain fog (Also due to candida)
- Visual difficulties
- Gastrointestinal disorders – bloating, gas, heartburn and indigestion.
- Skin problems such as persistent and chronic rashes.
- Indirectly lead to cancer due to free radicals and inflammation.
- Autoimmune diseases such as Hyperthyroidism, Multiple Sclerosis, Lupus, etc.
- Allergies
- Weight gain
- Hormonal issues
- Low libido, impotence
- Depression and anxiety
- Memory loss
- Dementia

Symptoms of Chronic Mercury Toxicity
Central Nervous System

- Irritability, anxiety/nervousness, often with difficulty in breathing
- Restlessness
- Exaggerated response to stimulation
- Fearfulness
- Emotional instability
  - Lack of self-control
  - Fits of anger, with violent, irrational behavior
- Loss of self-confidence, Indecision
- Shyness or timidity, being easily embarrassed
- Loss of memory, Inability to concentrate
- Lethargy/drowsiness
- Insomnia

4.4 Current methods of diagnosis

While there are many methods for diagnosing heavy metal poisoning, I have found the most accurate is through a hair analysis. Blood tests can detect it but only if the exposure was relatively recent. The toxins have to be in the blood at the time of the test. The problem is that the metals will eventually become stored in the soft tissues of the body as well as the organs and blood will not always detect it. In the clinic we prefer to do a thorough intake on the patient looking over their history of the illness, past possibilities of exposure combined with a hair analysis.

Times have changed and it is now relatively simple and inexpensive to get a hair analysis done. One of the best companies we have found is Great Plains Laboratory out of Lenexa, Kansas. Their website is **www.greatplainslaboratory.com.** Ask for the Heavy Metals Hair analysis. They can send you a kit which you will send back with a hair clipping. It can take a couple of weeks to get the results.

If you still would like to get a blood test done you can order it through Walk-In-Lab. As mentioned earlier, the website is **www.walkinlab.com.** The test is called the Heavy Metals Profile 2 Blood Test, test code #706200.

A relatively recent urine test has been developed which we use at the clinic. It is produced by Osumex at **www.osumex.us**. They also have a U.K. division.

There test is called the Heavy Metals Test General Kit. It is a simple urine test that can show you the results in about 20 minutes for exposure to mercury, lead, copper, manganese, nickel, cobalt and cadmium.

Of course, I always let patients know the above tests are best done by a qualified professional who can better interpret the results.

4.5 Conventional methods of treatment

Within the realm of conventional medicine, the standard treatment plan is to identify the particular heavy metal or chemicals. Once this is done then a series of chelating drugs are used and the process is monitored with 24 hour urine collection to test for the presence of the toxins. The drugs may be oral or done as intravenous EDTA chelation.

Conventional treatments may also use such procedures as suctioning the stomach, using the diuretic Mannitol, or steroid drugs as well as Hemodialysis if the kidneys are already failing.

The chelation drugs may be:

- Deferasirox (Exjade)– known side effects: renal (kidney failure), diarrhea, dizziness, nausea, stomach pain, voice changes, vomiting and death.
- Succimer (Chemet)– known side-effects: diarrhea, loose stools, loss of appetite, skin rash, chills and fever.
- Deferoxamine (Desferal) – known side-effects: bluish fingernails, lips or skin, blurred vision, convulsions, difficulty breathing, fast heartbeat, hearing problems and redness or flushing of the skin.
- Deferasirox (Jadenu) – known side-effects: agranulocytosis which can lead to serious infections and death. Also black tarry stools, chills, cough, fever, lower back or side pain, pale skin, sore throat, ulcers, sores or white spots in the mouth, unusual bleeding or bruising and unusual tiredness or weakness.
- Deferiprone (Ferriprox) – known side-effects: liver disease or weakened immune system.
- Trientine (Syprine) – known side-effects: unusually pale skin, unusual tiredness, fever, general feeling of discomfort, joint pain, skin rash, hives or blistering and swollen glands.

The above drugs are usually taken until no sign of the toxins are detected in the urine. This does not account for any still in the soft tissues.

4.6 Holistic treatment – The Heavy Metal Cleanse

If you read the above section on conventional treatments and their side-effects you may be ready to try a more holistic approach. I will cover those in this section as well as provide some wonderful case histories I have seen in my practice.

There are many herbs that work very well for chelating, or removing heavy metals from our bodies. As stated by The School of Natural Healing; **"Dr. Christopher liked bugleweed. His Heavy Mineral Bugleweed formula was his combination of choice whenever heavy metal poisoning was presented to him. He used these along with Epsom salt baths. One of his more dramatic cases was with a miner. Dr. Christopher had him take the Heavy Mineral Bugleweed formula with the Blood Stream formula, taking 3 hot baths with a pound of Epsom salts a week, spaced a day a part. After three weeks, that poor miner had to work hard to scrape dense, metallic grime off his bathtub. "**

The formula for the Bugleweed Heavy Metal Detox is actually quite simple as it consists of just Bugleweed, Yellow Dock and Lobelia.

The above protocol is usually followed for about three weeks. If any additional help is needed than let the body rest for a full week from the baths but continue with the formulas. Garlic is also found as a great adjunct to this treatment. In Dr. Paavo Airola book **The Miracle of Garlic** he relates the following regarding heavy metal poisoning and the use of garlic. "The threat to our health from environmental poisons, and specifically heavy metals, is increasing every day. Lead, mercury, cadmium, arsenic, and copper poisoning are becoming epidemic. Lead and mercury come mostly from polluted air plus industrial and medical uses, such as lead containing paint and mercury containing amalgam dental fillings. Contaminated fish are also a common source of mercury poisoning. Copper enters our bodies usually from copper water pipes, commonly used in plumbing."

I am including a standard heavy metal medication instructions for which I have seen wonderful success. The protocol requires taking the following holistic medications for a month or more.

1.) Liver and Gallbladder – 2 capsules 3 x a day, six days a week, one off.
2.) Heavy Metal Bugleweed Detox – 3 capsules 3 x a day, six days a week, one off.
3.) Milk Thistle – 2 dropperfuls 3 x a day, six days a week, one off.
4.) Blood Stream – 2 capsules 3 x a day, six days a week, one off.
5.) Vegan diet with extensive green drink juicing.

The **Liver and Gallbladder Formula** is used to aid in cleansing the liver as our main detox organ and it is required to be functioning well to aid in eliminating the chemicals from our systems. The herbs that compose the liver-gallbladder formula are: barberry, wild yam, cramp bark, fennel seed, ginger, catnip and peppermint.

The **Heavy Metal Bugleweed Detox**, as described above, is very useful in chelating the metals.

The **Blood Steam formula** aids the body in cleansing the blood as the metals are chelated out of the soft tissue sand enter the blood stream. The ingredients are Red clover blossoms, chaparral, licorice root, poke root, peach bark, Oregon grape root, stillingia, prickly ash bark, burdock root, and buckthorn bark.

We incorporate **Milk Thistle** due to it's well established ability to heal a damaged liver.

Now, how about some holistic treatments you can do in the house? A number of single herbs/procedures also do a great job with this condition.

- Dandelion is wonderful as it is a great liver cleanser.
- Red Clover is a superb blood cleanser.
- Stinging Nettle helps support the kidneys as they are working hard to eliminate the toxins via the urinary tract.
- Milk Thistle – As mentioned above.

- Cilantro as a great blood builder and cleanser.
- Saunas for sweating out the old to let in the new. It also increases circulation and blood flow.
- Zinc since most Americans are zinc deficient and it competes with cadmium and lead at the binding sites, thereby not allowing these toxic metals to remain in the system.
- Garlic as mention before. It also helps to protect against the damaging effects of the toxins. When rats were given garlic at the same time as cadmium and mercury, accumulation of the heavy metals in the liver, kidneys, bone, and testes was decreased and the activity of certain key enzymes was partially restored. In addition, cadmium excretion was increased.
- Chlorella significantly increased the urinary and fecal excretion of mercury while lowering it's levels in the brain and kidneys.
- Epsom salt baths are wonderful for pulling the toxins out through the skin.

As you can see, there are a variety of wonderful holistic medications and herbs for tackling this ever increasing problem in this society. But above all, please remember that diet, in both the short and long run, is a great way to chelate out the metals naturally as well as limiting any further exposure. My experience is a healthy vegan diet has been shown in clinical trials around the world to be an efficient method for not only curing this issue but limiting the exposure in the future.

CASE HISTORIES

I will be presenting here two case histories of patients I have worked with over the years, excerpted from my book, ***Case Histories From A Successful Naturopathic Clinic.***

Case History #1: Betsy.

One of the most prevalent conditions in America today as well as in other industrialized nations is heavy metal toxicity. It is found in the food, the air, the soil, cigarette smoking and in the cloths we wear. Pharmaceuticals are filled with them such as mercury, aluminum, cadmium, lead and arsenic.

Some time back a 47 year old female patient came into our clinic complaining of a number of autoimmune type reactions as well as a serious candida and mold infection. During her intake we found that she was a potter and sculptor who made extensive use of glazing. Heavy metals can be found in the clay itself as well as the chemicals used for glazing. Her home also had a very serious mold problem. Her blood work showed infections and a hair analysis showed extensive heavy metals as can be seen by the following lab result:

TOXIC METALS		RESULT mg/g	REFERENCE INTERVAL	PERCENTILE 68th 95th
Aluminum	(Al)	8.1	< 7.0	
Antimony	(Sb)	0.12	< 0.050	
Arsenic	(As)	0.048	< 0.060	
Barium	(Ba)	4.0	< 2.0	
Beryllium	(Be)	< 0.01	< 0.020	
Bismuth	(Bi)	0.096	< 2.0	
Cadmium	(Cd)	0.12	< 0.050	
Lead	(Pb)	5.6	< 0.60	
Mercury	(Hg)	0.15	< 0.80	
Platinum	(Pt)	< 0.003	< 0.005	
Thallium	(Tl)	< 0.001	< 0.002	
Thorium	(Th)	0.002	< 0.002	
Uranium	(U)	0.014	< 0.060	
Nickel	(Ni)	0.29	< 0.30	
Silver	(Ag)	5.5	< 0.15	
Tin	(Sn)	1.1	< 0.30	
Titanium	(Ti)	0.57	< 0.70	
Total Toxic Representation				

She was very high in Antimony, Barium, Lead, Nickel and Silver. These metals are notorious for wiping out the intestinal flora and bringing bout a severe candida overgrowth, thereby compromising the immune system. This left her open to so many other co-infections such as mold and other bacterial types. Her original presenting complaints included candida and hormonal imbalances.

We started her off with our standard candida cleanse, mentioned earlier in this document. This utilized a vegan diet due to it's low inflammatory nature and one low in natural sugar. She had to avoid all sugars and alcohol, even fruits for at least 18 days as well as use holistic medications for killing the candida, such as Black walnut and Pau'd Arco. We keep the bowels moving to help eliminate the dead yeast.

By the end of the 18 days she noticed a marked improvement in her thinking and level of energy. She proceeded to have the home cleaned out from the mold while we treated her for the mold in her lungs, again, using the above mold and yeast formulas, but at a much lower dosage and for several months. She remained on the vegan diet as it is well established that the fiber and anti-oxidants and other chemicals in the plants help chelate the heavy metals from her body.

At this time we also prescribed a natural heavy metal formula called Dr. Christopher's Bugle Heavy Metal Formula. It utilizes Bugleweed, a known herb with a very strong history of success for removing heavy metals from the body. She remained on this program for at least six months. As each month passed on the program she felt her health improving which we confirmed with blood work demonstrating the infections were disappearing. We finally ran another heavy metal hair test six months later. The surprising results are shown below:

		TOXIC METALS		PERCENTILE
		RESULT µg/g	REFERENCE INTERVAL	68th 95th
Aluminum	(Al)	3.6	< 7.0	
Antimony	(Sb)	0.035	< 0.050	
Arsenic	(As)	0.048	< 0.060	
Barium	(Ba)	1.5	< 2.0	
Beryllium	(Be)	< 0.01	< 0.020	
Bismuth	(Bi)	0.013	< 2.0	
Cadmium	(Cd)	0.046	< 0.050	
Lead	(Pb)	1.2	< 0.60	
Mercury	(Hg)	0.08	< 0.80	
Platinum	(Pt)	< 0.003	< 0.005	
Thallium	(Tl)	< 0.001	< 0.002	
Thorium	(Th)	0.001	< 0.002	
Uranium	(U)	0.020	< 0.060	
Nickel	(Ni)	0.12	< 0.30	
Silver	(Ag)	1.4	< 0.15	
Tin	(Sn)	0.14	< 0.30	
Titanium	(Ti)	0.34	< 0.70	
Total Toxic Representation				

As you can see from the above lab, the heavy metals showed a marked improvement which was mirrored in her improved energy levels, cognitive and memory abilities and a total lack of bronchial and sinus issues.

She remains vegan to this day and is a shining example of a healthy and happy individual. We are all very proud of her.

Case History #2: Samuel.

It is sad to me when a patient comes into the clinic after months or years of suffering due to the fact they were never properly diagnosed. Following is one such case.

Samuel was a 58 year old male who presented a rash from his head to his feet and had been suffering from it for the past nine months. The previous three months before we had our first appointment he had spent sitting in a chair or in bed as any movement caused it to flare up into an intense, maddening itch. He had gone to doctor after doctor including specialists such as dermatologist and even had skin punch biopsies done, to no avail for a diagnosis. His quality of life was at an all-time low and he had lost hope for a cure.

I went over his intake form and did what any good doctor would do and that is to try and find the root cause, not just treat the symptoms. I inquired as to what may have happened or changed in his life about nine or ten months ago. The only thing he could think of is that he had his mercury fillings removed just before the rash appeared. He described the procedure the dentist used. I discussed with the patient that the wrong procedure was done and that the mercury vapor had been inhaled and swallowed during the dental office visit.

Ingesting or inhaling mercury is like taking a massive dose of an antibiotic. It will destroy your bacterial micro-flora and leave you open to a massive candida overgrowth. I told him the rash was Candida Vasculitis, very common after such an event.

As with all of our chronic patients, the first thing we do is the 18 day candida cleanse. As mentioned earlier, this utilized a healthy, noninflammatory vegan diet with herbal medications such as Black Walnut and Pau'd Arco for eliminating the yeast. We also employ the use of Slippery Elm bark and Licorice root for soothing and healing the intestinal walls, so inflamed from the yeast overgrowth.

By the end of the 18 days, his body wide rash had shrunk to a small patch on his upper left arm. He stated he was feeling wonderful and his energy had much improved. I started him on a heavy metal detox using Dr. Christopher's Bugle Heavy Metal formula and he remained on the diet to allow his body a chance to heal while the chelation continued.

After a total of two months he no longer experienced any sign of the rashes and the detox was completed. He and his wife continued to be patients with the clinic for various other minor issues for a couple of years and the rash never made another appearance.

CHAPTER 5

HOW TO PREVENT THEIR RE-OCCURRENCE

OK, we managed to heal all of the above ills and can feel what a healthier body is meant to experience. Where do we go from here?

Sadly, our experience in a clinical environment tells us that most patients will eventually come and see us again over the years for the same or similar issue. This is due in large part to a return to the habits that brought about their condition in the first place.

While there are some common concerns to keep in mind for each of the three topics; Candida, Parasites and heavy Metal Toxicity, there are also a few unique concerns within each issue.

5.1 Diet as a major factor

I know from experience that this is not most patient's favorite subject, one of diet. As Doctor Christopher once stated, **"Talk to a friend about their diet and you will lose a friend"**. Sadly, I have seen this so many times. But it is a simple fact that you are what you eat and if you eat dead food it will not produce life within your body.

The scope of this subject is too large to be covered adequately so I will simply touch on some of the more important issues. Our new book on Curing Chronic Illness with a Raw, Vegan Diet will be released later this Fall.

As with all of our chronic patients, our initial goal is to get them on a full program utilizing a healthy, plant-based diet, monthly visits and taking the holistic medications as prescribed. Each program is unique to the patient but one of the common protocols, no matter the illness, is diet.

Our experience is that most folks are very misinformed about the health aspects of a plant-based diet. Fortunately, there has been an increasing number of studies verifying the health benefits:

"It is the position of the **American Dietetic Association** that appropriately planned vegetarian diets, including total vegetarian or vegan diets, are healthful, nutritionally adequate and may provide health benefits in the prevention and treatment of certain diseases"

From **The American Diabetes Association** "Is it safe for someone with diabetes to follow a vegetarian diet? Yes! A vegetarian diet is a healthy option, even if you have diabetes. Research supports that following this type of diet can help prevent and manage diabetes. In fact, research on vegan diets has found that carb and calorie restrictions were not necessary and still promoted weight loss and lowered participants' A1C".

The Dietitians of Canada Association: "Eating Guidelines for Vegans -Information about a Vegan Diet - A vegan eating pattern is based on grains, fruits, vegetables, legumes (dried beans, peas and lentils), seeds and nuts. It excludes meat, fish, poultry, dairy and eggs or products containing these foods and any other animal products. A vegan eating pattern has many potential health benefits. They include lower rates of obesity, heart disease, high blood pressure, type 2 diabetes and certain types of cancer. Other benefits include lower blood cholesterol levels and a lower risk for gallstones and intestinal problems."

In January, a report was published by the **EAT-Lancet Commission** on Food, Planet, Health, the result of 37 scientists from around the globe who teamed up to determine how diet impacts the environment.

The scientists concluded that the way we currently eat is unsustainable, and we would have to drastically cut back on animal products and shift to almost entirely plant foods in order to sustainably feed an expected population of 10 billion people in 2050.

The world's largest organization of food and nutrition professionals has announced its position on plant-based diets - and deemed them 'appropriate for all stages of the life cycle, including pregnancy, lactation, infancy, childhood, adolescence, older adulthood, and for athletes. By doing so, **The Academy of Nutrition and Dietetics** has sent a powerful message about the universal suitability of vegan diets - breaking down perhaps one of the last standing misconceptions of plant-based eating.

In 2010, **The United Nations** published a report, Assessing the Environmental Impacts of Consumption and Production, in which they concluded that meaningfully reducing agriculture's contribution to global food insecurity and climate change "would only be possible with a substantial **worldwide diet change, away from animal products.**"

In late 2017, the **World Wildlife Fund**— now the World Wildlife Fund for Nature— published a report, *Appetite for Destruction,* focused on the **devastating impacts of meat and dairy production to wildlife species** and ecosystems. The report says animal product consumption is responsible for 60 per cent of all biodiversity loss, in large part due to the **clearing of land to grow crops for animal feed.** The report urges consumers to "Eat more plants," and "Moderate your meat consumption, both red and white. Enjoy other sources of proteins such as peas, beans and nuts instead."

As can be seen, a large number of science based organizations back the validity of a healthy plant-based diet. Now please do not get me wrong, being vegan is not enough. You may note that I keep writing about a "Healthy vegan diet". When I went vegetarian back in 1981 and vegan in 1991 there was a website called **veganessentials.com**. At that time (in the 1990's) it had maybe 50 or so items. Now there are over 1500 items meant to meet your most wide spread plant-based cravings. From one perspective I think this is wonderful as new comers to the vegan lifestyle can be over-whelmed as to what food choices and substitutes they can find. Many automatically think life as a vegan is carrots and cabbage. Websites like theirs show there are now more options than ever before.

But this can also come with an unhealthy price tag. These foods are at best, meant to be treats or as transition foods. This can enable people to begin to change their eating habits without giving up "the foods they love". Unfortunately, some folks let these "snacks" become their main diet and this can have some serious health problems. Just like with the average junk food, these are not meant to be in a wholesome diet, in the long run.

So what can you eat? As Doctor Christopher stated; "**A diet rich in fruits and vegetables, nuts, grains and seeds**." This is also best in the wholesome natural state. It has been shown that a plant based diet will supply you with all of the protein, carbs, vitamins and minerals you need. Also, the fresher and less processed the foods the more enzyme activity will be present which than enables your body not to need to use its own store.

As I stated this is too broad a subject for this book. There are wonderful books and documentaries out now that can supply you with plenty of sound nutritional advice. As stated earlier, this Fall we will also be coming out with our book for treating chronic diseases with diet. Please consider watching such plant-based documentaries as: **Forks Over Knives**, **Veducated**, **Simply Raw: Reversing Diabetes in 30 days**, **Fat, Sick and Nearly Dead**, **What the Health**, and **Pure Plant Nation**.

So, in short: improve Your Diet
- Maximize your health by eating whole, organic foods. Eating a healthy diet is key to nourishing and rebuilding your body.
- Eat whole, organic unprocessed foods.
- Eat local in-season foods whenever possible.
- Include cultured and fermented foods in your diet.
- Include healthy fats in your diet.
- Eat one-third of your food raw.

Following is a very simple one day menu plan:

Vegan Outreach Meal Plan - 2300 calories Single Day Report

Meal Plan by Dina Aronson, MS, RD

Date: Monday

PCF Ratio

Carbs (53%) Protein (15%) Fat (32%)

Breakfast	Serving Size	Gram Wt.	Calories (kcal)	Protein (g)	Carbs (g)	Fat (g)	Sat fat (g)	Trans Fat (g)	Omega-3 (g)	Dietary Fiber (g)
Scrambled Tofu	1 serving	470	268	20	20	13	2	0	0	5
WHOLE WHEAT BREAD, CP	2 slices	56	138	5	26	2	1	0	0	4
CANTALOUPE, RAW	2 medium wedge	138	48	1	12	0	0	0	0	1
MARGARINE SPREAD, TUB	1 tbsp	14	75	0	0	9	0	0	0	0
Meal Total:		678	529	27	57	25	3	0	0	10
Morning Snack										
SOY YOGURT, VANILLA	6 oz	170	150	5	26	3	0	0	0	0
FLAX SEED	2 tbsp	24	118	5	8	8	1	0	4	7
Meal Total:		194	268	10	34	11	1	0	4	7
Lunch										
Black Bean and Sweet Potato Salad	1.5 servings	658	509	18	81	12	0	0	0	18
GRAPEFRUIT, RAW	1 fruit	246	91	1	24	0	0	0	0	0
Meal Total:		904	600	19	105	12	0	0	0	18
Afternoon Snack										
TRAIL MIX SNACK, REGULAR	2 oz	57	262	8	25	17	3	0	0	0
Meal Total:		57	262	8	25	17	3	0	0	0
Dinner										
QUINOA COOKED	1.5 cups	360	384	18	51	12	0	0	0	12
Grilled vegetables	1 servings	442	195	6	30	8	1	0	0	8
Meal Total:		802	579	24	81	20	1	0	0	20

Evening Snack

Vegan Outreach Meal Plan - 2300 calories Single Day Report (continued)

	Serving Size	Gram Wt.	Calories (kcal)	Protein (g)	Carbs (g)	Fat (g)	Sat fat (g)	Trans Fat (g)	Omega-3 (g)	Dietary Fiber (g)
Evening Snack										
FRUIT SALAD, WATER PACK	1 cup	245	74	1	19	0	0	0	0	2
Meal Total:		245	74	1	19	0	0	0	0	2
Daily Total:		2,880	2,312	88	322	86	8	0	5	57

	Folate (mcg)	Vit B-12 (mcg)	Vit-C (mg)	Vit-E IU (IU)	Calcium (mg)	Iron (mg)	Magnesium (mg)	Potassium (mg)	Sodium (mg)	Zinc (mg)
Breakfast										
Scrambled Tofu	70	0	163	3	142	5	95	1,081	819	2
WHOLE WHEAT BREAD, CP	28	0	0	1	40	2	48	141	295	1
CANTALOUPE, RAW	23	0	58	0	15	0	15	426	12	0
MARGARINE SPREAD, TUB	0	0	0	0	0	0	0	0	75	0
Meal Total:	121	0	221	4	198	7	158	1,648	1,202	4
Morning Snack										
SOY YOGURT, VANILLA	0	0	0	0	0	0	0	0	25	0
FLAX SEED	67	0	0	2	48	1	87	163	8	1
Meal Total:	67	0	0	2	48	1	87	163	33	1
Lunch										
Black Bean and Sweet Potato Salad	42	0	91	1	166	8	47	710	1,002	0
GRAPEFRUIT, RAW	30	0	94	0	27	0	22	362	2	0
Meal Total:	72	0	185	1	193	8	69	1,072	1,005	1
Afternoon Snack										
TRAIL MIX SNACK, REGULAR	40	0	1	0	44	2	90	388	130	2
Meal Total:	40	0	1	0	44	2	90	388	130	2
Dinner										
QUINOA COOKED	48	0	0	9	45	6	192	780	18	7
Grilled vegetables	71	0	60	0	41	2	51	1,202	188	1
Meal Total:	119	0	60	9	86	8	243	1,982	206	8
Evening Snack										
FRUIT SALAD, WATER PACK	7	0	5	0	17	1	12	191	7	0
Meal Total:	7	0	5	0	17	1	12	191	7	0
Daily Total:	426	0	472	16	585	27	659	5,445	2,582	15

5.2 Lifestyle choices

So, as we finish this book, I would like to cover a few things we can do to help avoid the re-occurrence of the previous issues.

PURIFY YOUR WATER:

The average person's tap water likely contains traces of chlorine, fluoride, calcium, magnesium, sodium, sulfates, and more! In addition those, there are more serious substances such as iron, manganese, copper, aluminum, and other chemicals.

HEAVY METAL TESTING:

Make sure to have yourself tested at least once a year. Sadly, in the world we live in this has become a necessity.

Drink 6 to 8 glasses of filtered or purified water daily.

Use a dry brush to get the lymphatic system working on the legs after showering.

Get rid of all plastic containers and water bottles made from BPA plastic. BPA found in many plastic containers is considered to be an endocrine disruptor or xenoestrogen, a class of compounds that can suppress male hormones and mimic female hormones by binding with estrogen receptors. I opt for stainless steel and glass containers and use glassware instead of plastic.

Remove mercury fillings if possible through a special Integrative Medical Dentist so that the mercury was not drawn into the brain or organs.

Get rid of all pots and pans that are Teflon-coated or aluminum.

Use glass, carbon steel, titanium, and enamel cookware. Both aluminum and non-stick cookware are well known for their toxic dangers, and stainless steel can expose you to carcinogenic nickel.

Avoid smoking and second hand smoke as it causes cadmium poisoning.

Make sure you purchase your natural herbal remedies from a reputable source with strict quality testing. Some colloidal silvers can lead to silver poisoning, and some folk remedies can be high in mercury, lead and arsenic, either due to alleged medicinal properties or through unintentional contamination.

Avoid cosmetics with aluminum bases, mineral powders that contain bismuth, and aluminum-laden antiperspirants, which have been shown to increase your Alzheimer's risk by as much as 300 percent!

Avoid vaccinations that inject mercury or aluminum directly into your bloodstream.

Wear masks and protective clothing if you work around heavy metals

Increase your fiber intake with a healthy balance of soluble and insoluble fiber.

Drink plenty of purified water, at least half your body weight in ounces each day. (For example, a 120-pound person would require 60 ounces of water, or seven tall glasses.)

Washing conventionally grown, raw vegetables and fruits with a suitable, natural disinfectant solution that is fit for consumption. Salt water may also be helpful to some extent. Clean running water should be used for rinsing.

Avoid antibiotics when it is safe to do so.

CLOSING THOUGHTS:

As the saying goes, the best defense is a good offense. Choose to live a healthy lifestyle rich in exercise, fresh air, sunshine, lots of fresh fruits and vegetables and their juices and as much of a stress-free life as you can. Take up yoga (good for the moving the lymphatic system), take walks, find meaning-full friendships, not just social media ones. Do what type of job makes you happy and not just for riches. A rich life is defined by the joy and love in your heart, not simply the size of your bank account or the number of "friends" on Facebook and such. I have come to learn the true law in a healing program is:

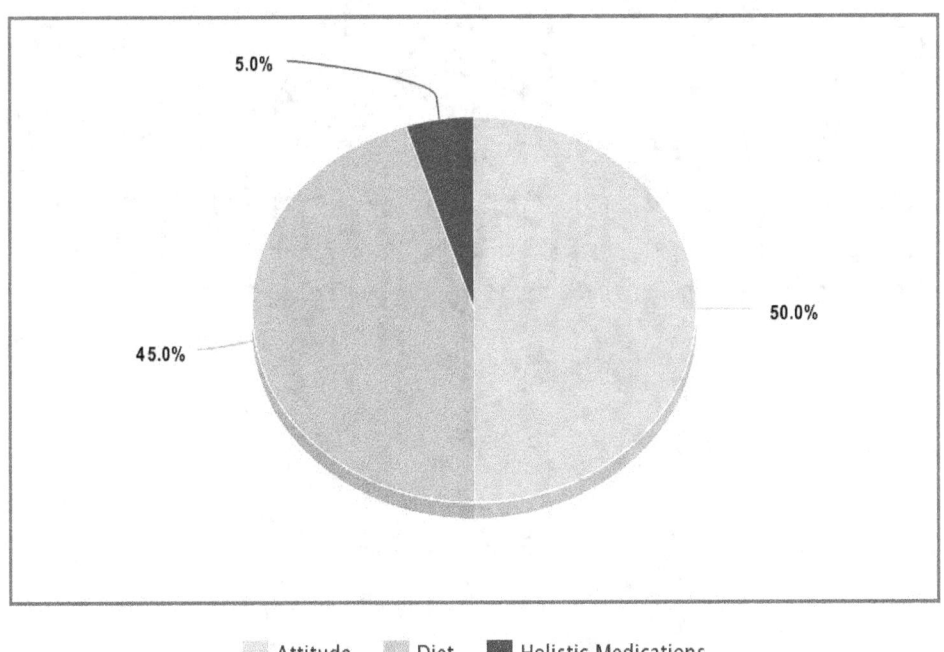

A Law Of Healing
Dr. Earendil Spindelilus

PART TWO – HOLISTIC FIRST-AID

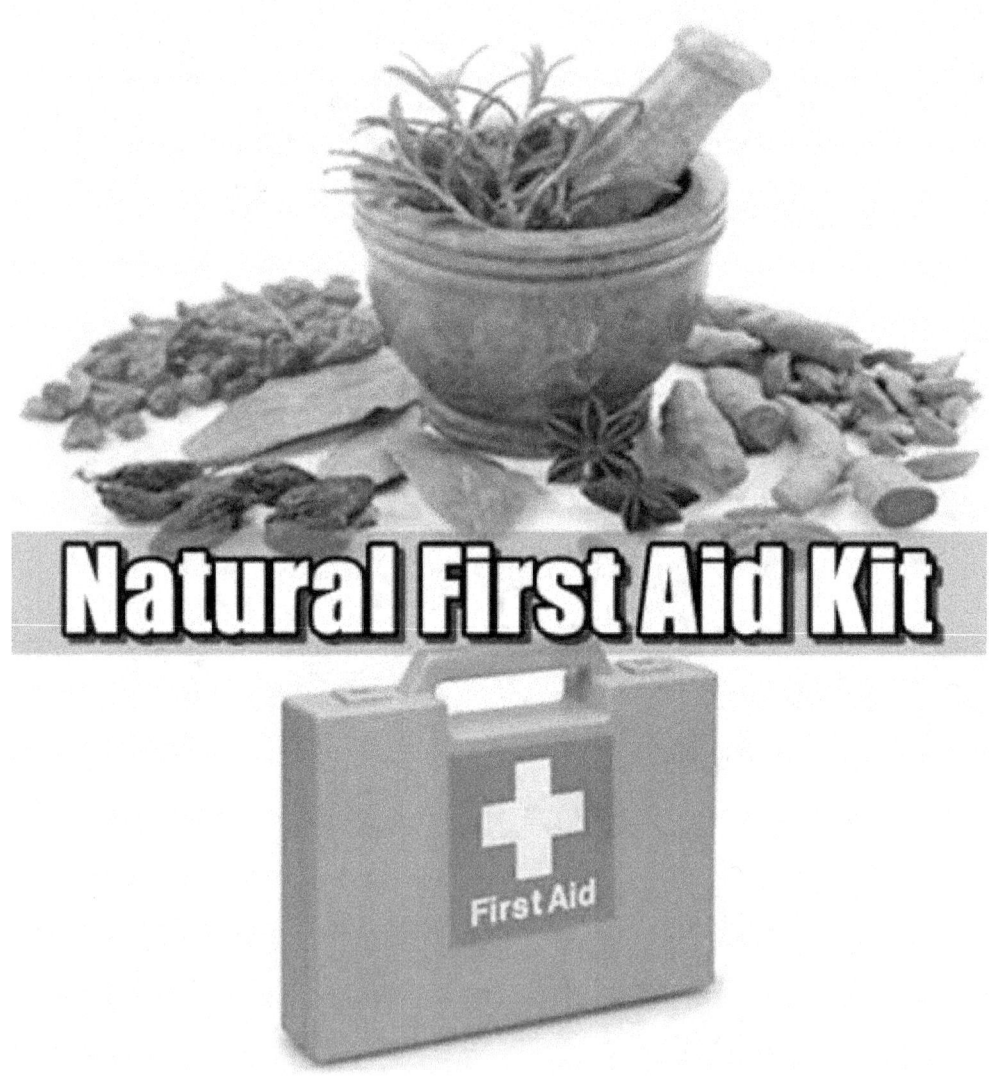

CHAPTER 6

Introduction

"An Herbalist in every home and a Master Herbalist in every community"
Dr. John R. Christopher

I can say that while technology seems to have made lives easier, I would not say it has made them better. A case in point is the lack of knowledge these days in the proper care and feeding of emergency situations. There was a time when most folks had at least a rudimentary understanding of first aid care and could handle most situations on their own. Most families or villages had a skilled healer in the community who knew enough to intervene when an accident occurred.

Sadly, this is not the case in today's world. Very few have even the basic knowledge of how to treat an open wound or a snake bite, let along a broken bone or a heart attack. Hospitals are now overrun with "emergencies" that in the past would never have even required the attention of a doctor. A few years back four separate hospitals closed their doors in one year in Los Angeles due to excessive use of the emergency room trauma centers. Patients who truly needed the ER would not be able to get treatment due to the lack of care as the hospitals were overrun with non life threatening situations.

According to the theguardian.com: "Up to 150,000 people a year could be dying unnecessarily because first aid is not widely enough known, a charity warns today. Situations where first aid could potentially make a difference include suffocations due to blocked airways, which claim 2,500 lives every year, and heart attacks, which kill 29,000.

St John Ambulance launched a new campaign to get more people to learn first aid skills. Its survey of more than 2,000 people found that 59% would not feel confident trying to save a life.

Meanwhile, almost a quarter (24%) would do nothing if they saw somebody struggling and would either wait for an ambulance to arrive or hope that a passerby knew first aid."

Curad, maker of adhesive bandages, in conjunction with the American Safety & Health Institute (ASHI), surveyed 200 first aid trainers concerning the general public's knowledge and preparedness when it comes to first aid. "When faced with a first aid emergency--no matter how minor or severe--our members say the biggest mistake people make is that they panic," indicates paramedic Ralph Shenefelt, general manager of ASHI. "By learning basic first aid and having the proper supplies to deal with minor first aid situations, the panic factor could be eased dramatically.

According to Wikipedia: "Skills of what is now known as first aid have been recorded throughout history, especially in relation to warfare, where the care of both traumatic and medical cases is required in particularly large numbers. The bandaging of battle wounds is shown on Classical Greek pottery from c. 500 BC, whilst the parable of the Good Samaritan includes references to binding or dressing wounds. There are numerous references to first aid performed within the Roman army, with a system of first aid supported by surgeons, field ambulances, and hospitals. Roman legions had the specific role of capsarii, who were responsible for first aid such as bandaging, and are the forerunners of the modern combat medic. Further examples occur through history, still mostly related to battle, with examples such as the Knights Hospitaller in the 11th century AD, providing care to pilgrims and knights in the Holy Land.

With technology comes more dependence on it's gifts and as can be seen from above, thousands are needlessly dying simply due to a lack of knowledge about basic first-aid skills. This is where this books come in. Not only will we be covering how to administer first-aid in a variety of situations, we will also be learning how this can be done in a more holistic, natural manner.

In this book we will learn about the natural treatment for such issues as burns, bleeding both minor and more severe, various types of poisonings, broken bone after care, snake bites, immediate life saving care for a heart attack or stroke victim, eye injuries, minor dental complaints and many more.

I will also be giving case histories where these tools have been used successfully, both on our clinic as well as from our patients who were taught these simple, historically proven techniques.

As always, please keep in mind that the care of a professional health care provider is sometimes required and we do not want you to make medical decisions on your own that may jeopardize yours or another life.

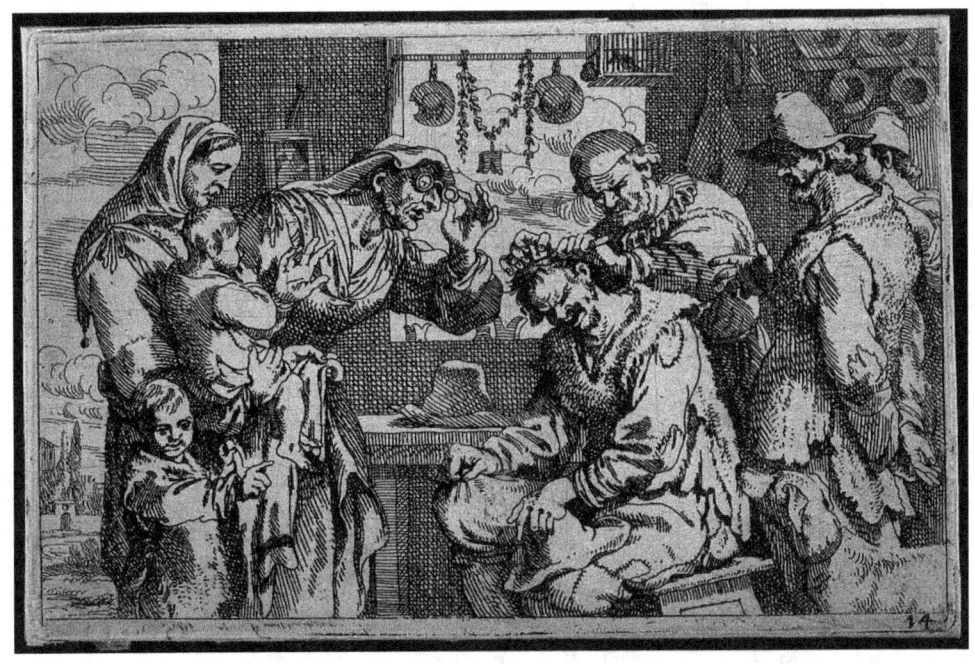

CHAPTER 7

BASIC FIRST-AID

7.1 Burns

This has to be one of the most common issues we have treated in the clinic as well as from family and friends. This can range for something as simple as a first degree sunburn to third degree house fires and electrical burns.

The American Burn Association states that:
- 44 percent of all admissions to burn centers result from fire or flame burns.
- 33 percent of all burn center admissions result from scalding injuries caused by wet or moist heat.
- Direct contact with a hot source accounts for nine percent of burn center admissions.
- Electrical burns account for four percent of burn center admissions.
- Chemical burns account for three percent of all burn center admissions.
- The remaining seven percent of burn center admissions are caused by other, miscellaneous sources.

The American Burn Association reports the following pediatric burn statistics for 2000:
- Scalding is the most common burn injury in children under four years old, accounting for 200,000 injuries per year.
- An estimated 50 percent of scalds are from spilled food and drinks, while the remainder are primarily from hot tap water and hot objects such as irons, stoves, and heaters.
- Each year, roughly 250,000 children under age 17 require medical attention for burn injuries.
- Roughly 15,000 children require hospitalization for burn injuries.

- About 1,100 children per year die from fires and burn injuries.

The American Burn Association states that of the 3,400 U.S. burn injury deaths each year:
- 2,550 of these deaths are a result of residential fires.
- 300 of these deaths result from vehicle crash fires.
- The remaining 550 result from other causes, such as flames, smoke inhalation, scalding, and electricity.

And finally ...

The Centers for Disease Control and Prevention provides the following statistics for costs related to burns:
- Males account for roughly $4.8 billion, or 64 percent, or total fire and burn-related costs each year, while females account for the remaining $2.7 billion, or 36 percent.
- Fatal burn and fire injuries cost roughly $3 billion, which accounts for two percent of the total cost of fatal injuries.
- Burn and fire hospitalization accounts for $1 billion, or one percent of hospitalized injury costs.
- Non-hospitalized burn and fire injuries account for two percent of non-hospitalized injury costs, or $3 billion.

As can be seen from the above statistics, so much of this could be avoided if we knew how to care for our own injuries. Of course, this does not negate the fact that there are times we would need the care of a qualified healthcare provider. This section is for those who do not have access to a hospital or another doctor.

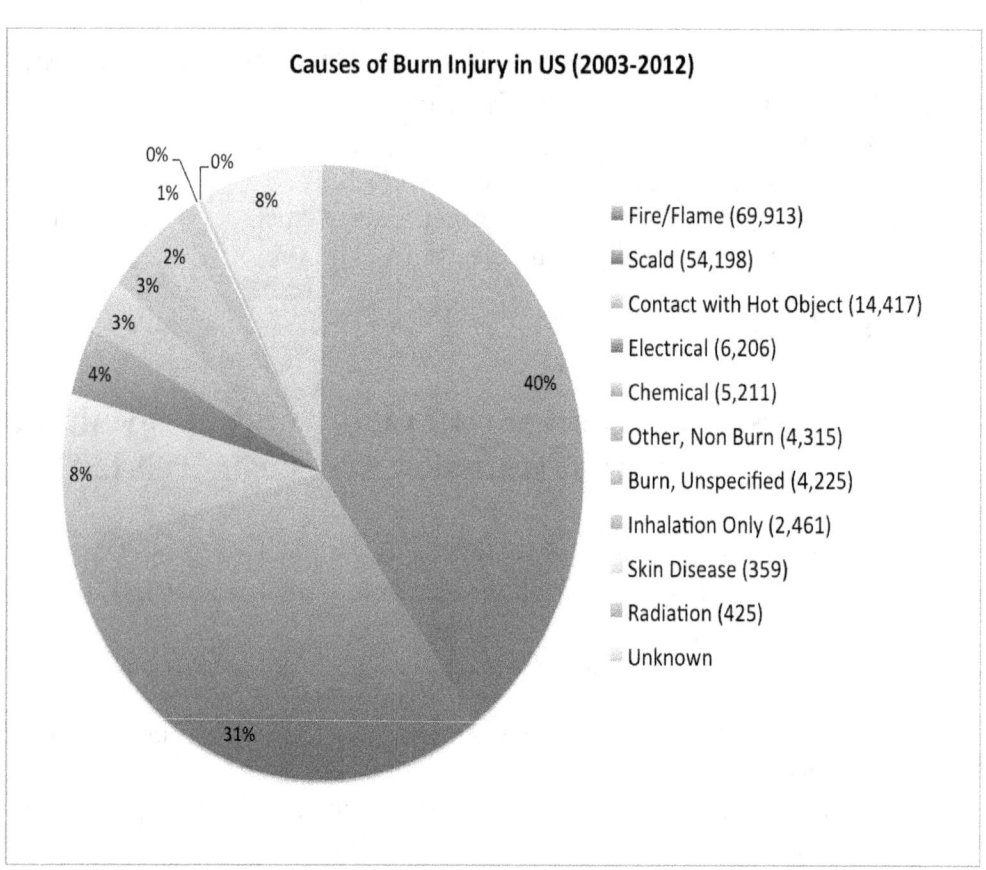

The good news is that there are wonderful history proven protocols that we can do to care for our injuries with natural holistic medicines. I will go over the varying degrees of burns, their types and the basic first aid for treating during an emergency.

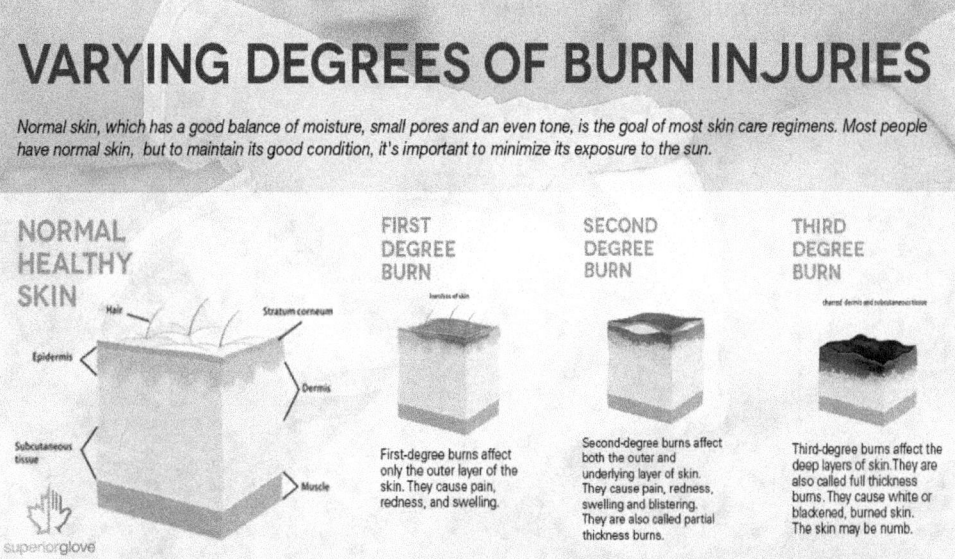

The above chart shows most burns are classified as first through third degree. There are higher classifications but that is beyond the scope of this book and they do REQUIRE a professionals assistance.

Types of first degree burns:

First-degree burns cause minimal skin damage. They are also called "superficial burns" because they affect the outermost layer of skin. Signs of a first-degree burn include:

- redness
- minor inflammation, or swelling
- pain
- dry, peeling skin occurs as the burn heals

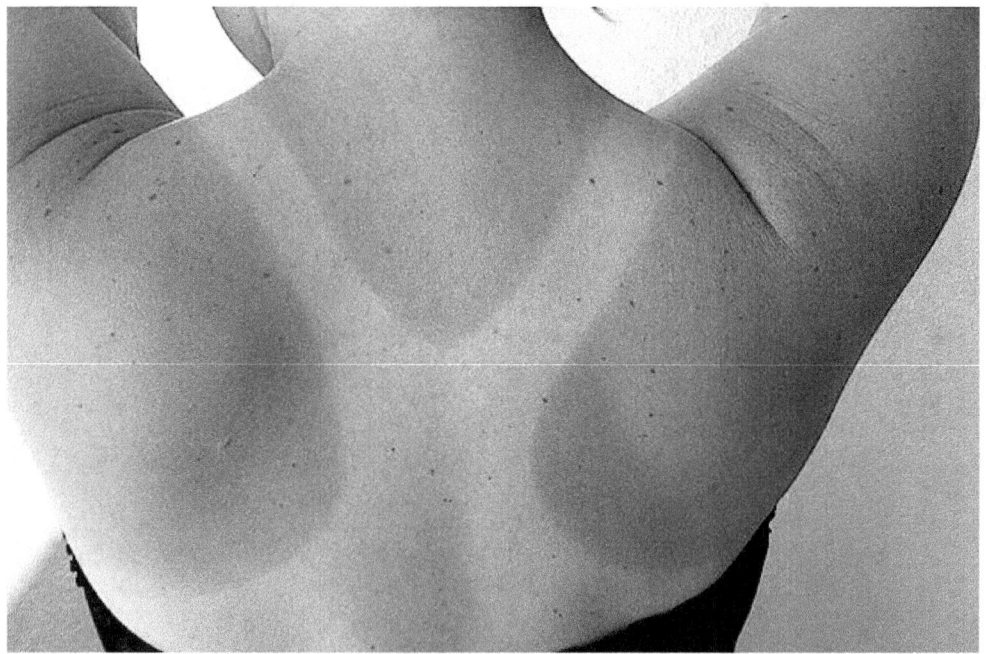

This burn affects only the top layer of skin, the signs and symptoms disappear once the skin cells shed. First-degree burns usually heal within 7 to 10 days without scarring.

CARE FOR FIRST DEGREE BURN:

The first thing you can do is to soak the burn in cool water. For pain and to aid in healing, the tried and true method used by most patients is a gel made from Aloe Vera. You can make this yourself from the fresh leaves of the plant or you can obtain the gels easily from most health food and pharmacy stores over the counter. Make sure NOT to use ice as this can make the damage worse. Do not use cotton balls as the fibers can stick to the burn possibly leading to infection.

Types of Second degree burns:

Second-degree burns are more serious because the damage extends beyond the top layer of skin. This type of burn causes the skin to blister and become extremely red and sore.

Some blisters pop open, giving the burn a wet or weeping appearance. Over time, thick, soft, scab-like tissue called fibrinous exudate may develop over the wound.

Due to the delicate nature of these wounds, keeping the area clean and bandaging it properly is required to prevent infection. This also helps the burn heal more quickly. As with first-degree burns, avoid cotton balls. Some second-degree burns take longer than three weeks to heal, but most heal within two to three weeks without scarring, but often with pigment changes to the skin.

Second Degree Burns

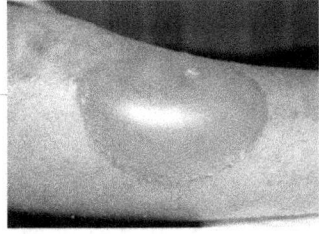

- Partial Thickness Burn
- Burns Epidermis and Dermis
- *Blisters forming is the key to DX*
- Mottled, Swelling, Wet, and Painful
- 3-4 Weeks to heal
- Cause Excessive Exposure to Sun, Radiation, Hot or Boiling Liquids, or Fire

CARE FOR SECOND DEGREE BURN:

To treat for this type of burn run it under cool water for 15 minutes or more. Aloe Vera will work with this type of burn but infection becomes a greater possibility so we opt for a preparation that is more effective at fighting a possible infection and does wonders for lowering the risk for scarring. This is a famous formula designed by Dr. Christopher and is called the burn ointment:

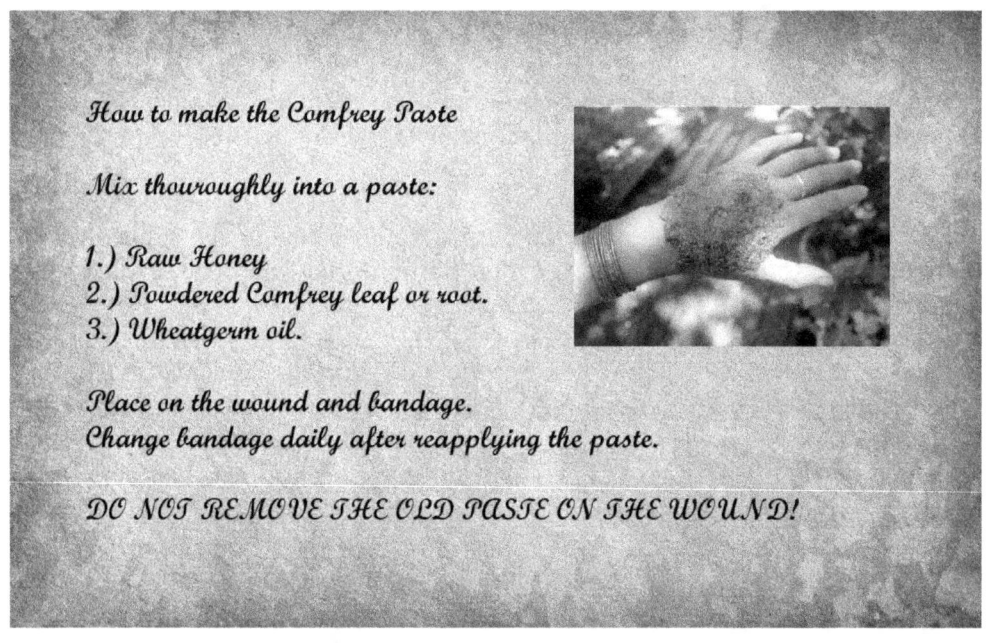

How to make the Comfrey Paste

Mix thouroughly into a paste:

1.) Raw Honey
2.) Powdered Comfrey leaf or root.
3.) Wheatgerm oil.

Place on the wound and bandage.
Change bandage daily after reapplying the paste.

DO NOT REMOVE THE OLD PASTE ON THE WOUND!

This is a very simple formula that has been used successfully for over 60 years. I have personally seen this remarkable mixture heal very serious burns with no scarring afterwards.

As you will notice, the main herb is Comfrey. As Dr. Christopher defined it, "Comfrey is one of the patriarchal herbs that I believe harkens back to the Garden of Eden. The Creator placed it on the Earth knowing that the human race was going to make a rough time of it and would need a universal salve for the wounds of war."

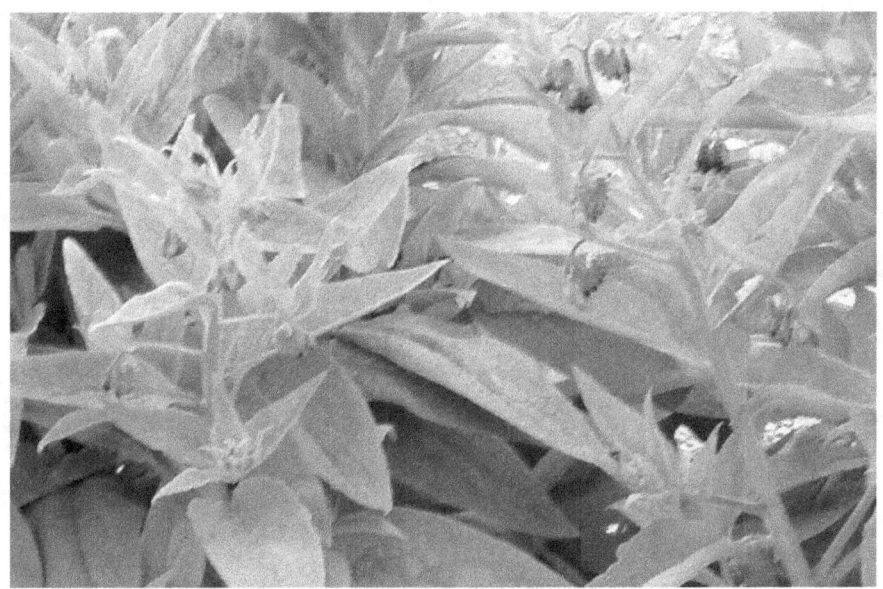

COMFREY

One of the most amazing properties of Comfrey is it's ability as a cell proliferate. This means that is able to cause cells to regrow very quickly. I have seen patient's broken arms heal in a third to half the time it commonly takes.

Some of the benefits of Comfrey include:

- Accelerate Wound Healing
- Relieves Back Pain
- Hydrates and repairs skin
- Boosts bone healthcare

For those who have read my book titled *Case Histories From A Successful Naturopathic Clinic,* you may remember the case of patient who had an advanced case of gangrene on his foot and was at a high risk for amputation. One of the main herbal formulas used contained a significant amount of Comfrey in it and the results were amazing. His foot, which had seriously decayed by the time he called (two months), completely regrew the flesh and muscle and left very little scar after months of treatment. Below are the before and after pictures. Please be aware the before is somewhat graphic.

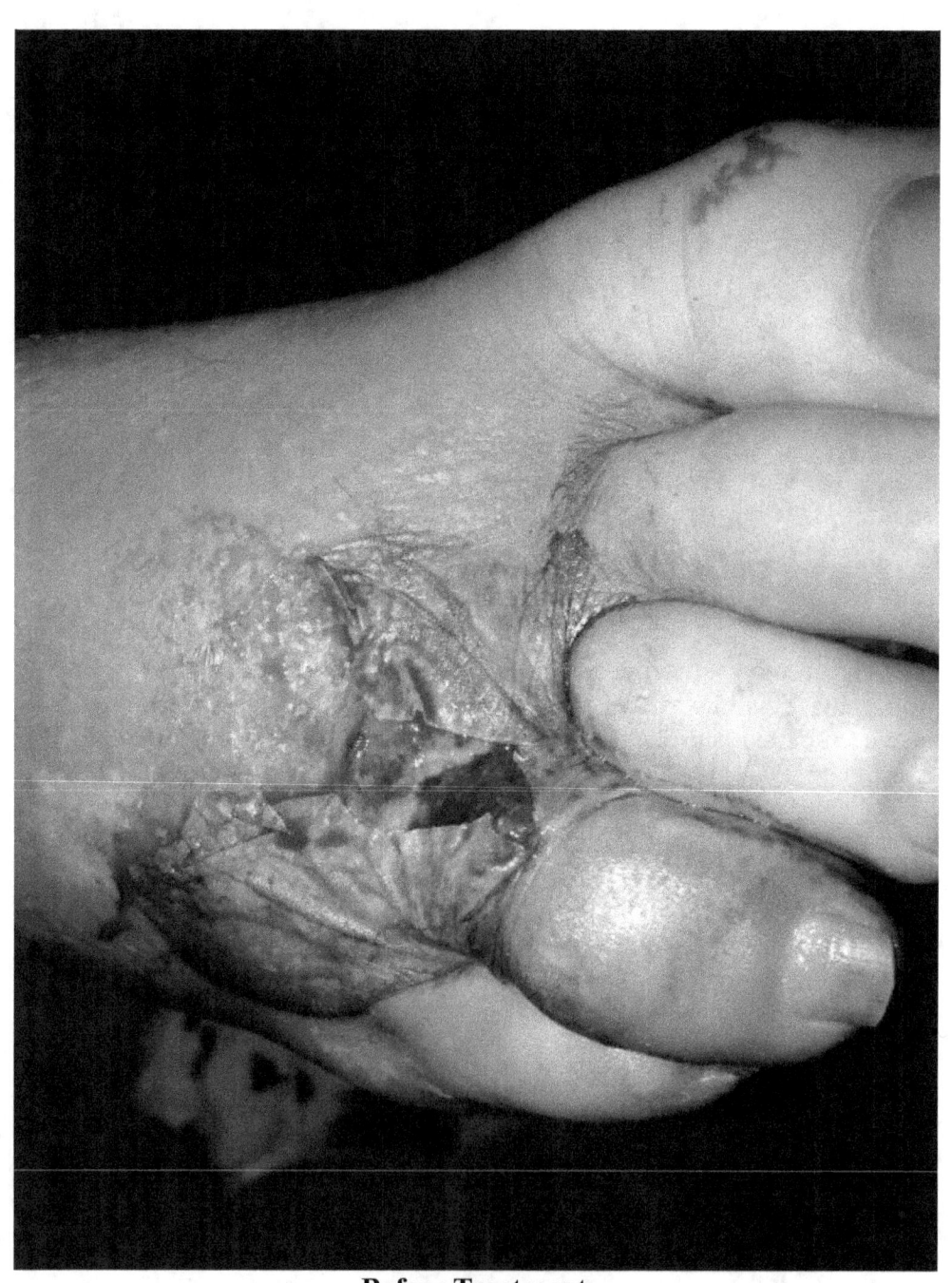
Before Treatment

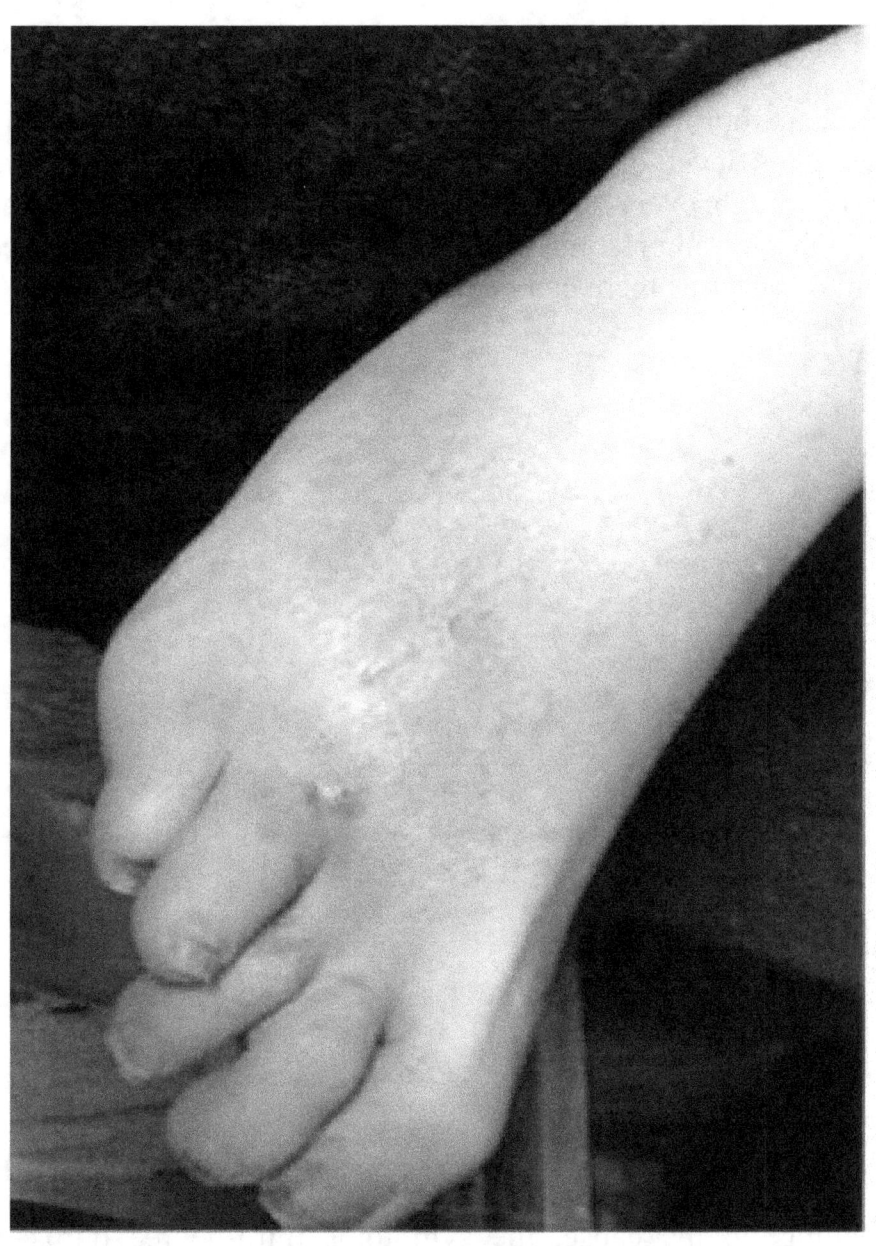

After several months of treatment

Types of Third degree burns:

Other than fourth degree burns, third degree burns are the most severe. This level of burn includes the most damage and may extend through every layer of skin. Risk of infection is usually very high. An interesting note is that these are often the least painful of burns as there can be extensive nerve damage.

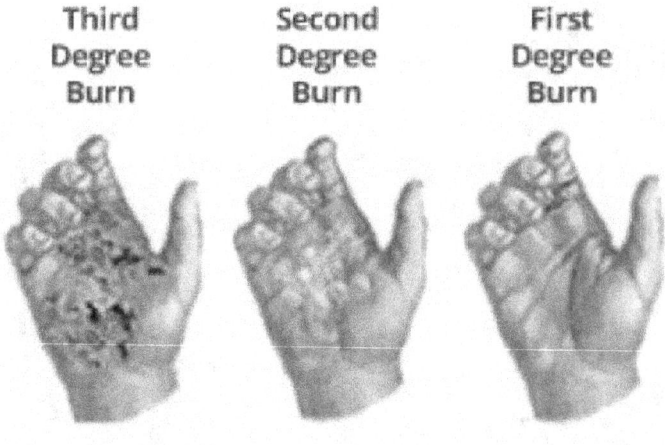

Depending on the cause, the symptoms third-degree burns can exhibit include:

- waxy and white color
- charring

- dark brown color
- raised and leathery texture
- blisters that do not develop

Without surgery, these wounds heal with severe scarring and contracture (where the limbs, fingers and such heal in a deformed manner and are not able to fully extend). While there is no set timeline for complete spontaneous healing for third-degree burns, we have seen healing occur more rapidly when holistic protocols are utilized.

As I discussed earlier, this can be a very serious burn and professional care is recommended. This book is for those who may not have easy access to a qualified healthcare provider. If you must treat it yourself then we find the Comfrey Paste formula or the B, F and C formula very effective. We would treat it by thickly coating the burn area with the paste or salve and wrapping it. It needs to be changed at least once a day as the body will absorb quite a bit of the salve. DO NOT remove the salve left over each time you change it. Simply reapply more salve on top of the old. You can also treat each day for possible infection by making sure the patient took either Dr. Christopher's Infection Formula at 4 capsules five times a day or by taking Garlic capsules at the same dosage. This may take weeks for the burn to heal, usually with little to no scarring.

7.2 Rashes

A rash is defined by Wikipedia as: A change of the human skin which affects its color, appearance, or texture. A rash may be localized in one part of the body, or affect all the skin. Rashes may cause the skin to change color, itch, become warm, bumpy, chapped, dry, cracked or blistered, swell, and may be painful.

The causes, and therefore treatments for rashes, vary widely. Diagnosis must take into account such things as the appearance of the rash, other symptoms, what the patient may have been exposed to, occupation, and occurrence in family members. The diagnosis may confirm any number of conditions. The presence of a rash may aid diagnosis; associated signs and symptoms are diagnostic of certain diseases. For example, the rash in measles is an erythematous, morbilliform, maculopapular rash that begins a few days after the fever starts. It classically starts at the head, and spreads downwards.

Skin rash facts
- *Rash* is not a specific diagnosis. Instead it refers to any sort of inflammation and/or discoloration that distorts the skin's normal appearance.
- Common rashes include eczema, poison ivy, hives, and athlete's foot.
- Infections that cause rashes may be fungal, bacterial, parasitic, or viral.
- Over-the-counter products may be helpful treatments for many skin rashes.
- Rashes lasting more than a few days that are unexplained should be evaluated by a doctor.

Some of the more common types of rashes:

Atopic dermatitis
- Seborrheic dermatitis
- Contact dermatitis
- Diaper rash
- Stasis dermatitis

- Psoriasis
- Hives
- Nummular eczema
- Drug eruptions
- Heat rash (miliaria)

Psoriasis is an autoimmune disorder and is therefore beyond the scope of this book. Please check out my book *Case Histories of a Successful Naturopathic Clinic* for more information.

Most of the rashes above fall within the realm of allergic reactions and yeast and fungus. I will cover in this section how to treat those conditions.

Allergy Type Rashes:

Let's start with **allergic** types of rashes. These are very common and are often very simple to treat. As a Naturopath it is my inclination to treat the root cause (meaning why are you allergic to something in the first place) but the scope of this book is mainly for first aid treatments.

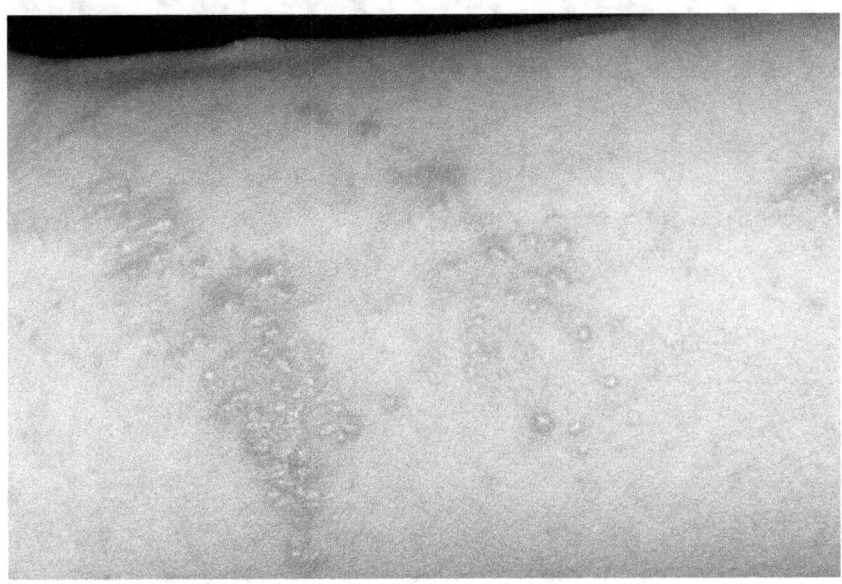

Poison Oak

One of the most common types of allergic rashes are contact dermatitis. Contact dermatitis is a rash that is brought on either by contact with a specific chemical to which the patient is uniquely allergic or with a substance that directly irritates the skin. Some chemicals are both irritants and allergens. This rash tends to be weepy and oozy and affects the parts of the skin which have come in direct contact with the offending substance. Common examples of allergic contact dermatitis are poison ivy, poison sumac, poison oak (same chemical, different plant) and reactions to costume jewelry containing nickel.

We use two different herbal aids to treat both the itch and the rash itself. The first is something we call Green Salve. It is made from a combination of Comfrey, Chickweed and Plantain. Many years ago this was a school project of mine and it was found to be so effective we continue to use it to this day in the clinic. It is made with equal parts of each of the herbs in an olive oil and bees wax base.

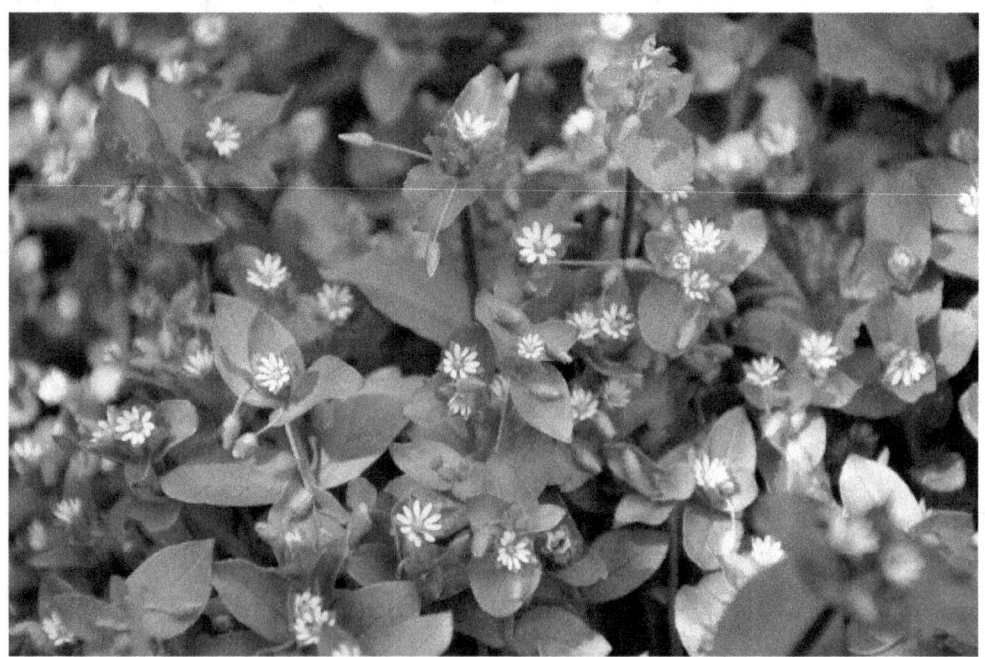

Chickweed (Stellaria Media)

We discussed earlier that Comfrey is a wonderful cell proliferate, meaning it has the ability to cause cells to regrow quickly. Chickweed has a wonderful reputation for soothing skin irritations.

Some of the benefits of Chickweed include:

- Prevents inflammation
- Encourages weight loss
- Alleviates respiratory problems
- Speeds up healing

Plantain:

There are two types of Plantain and both have similar properties and can be used interchangeably:

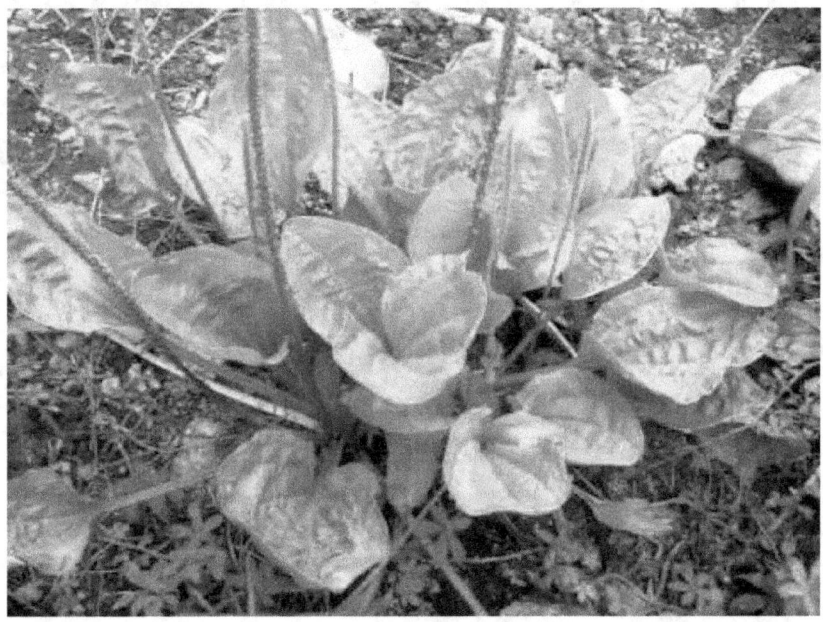

Plantago Major

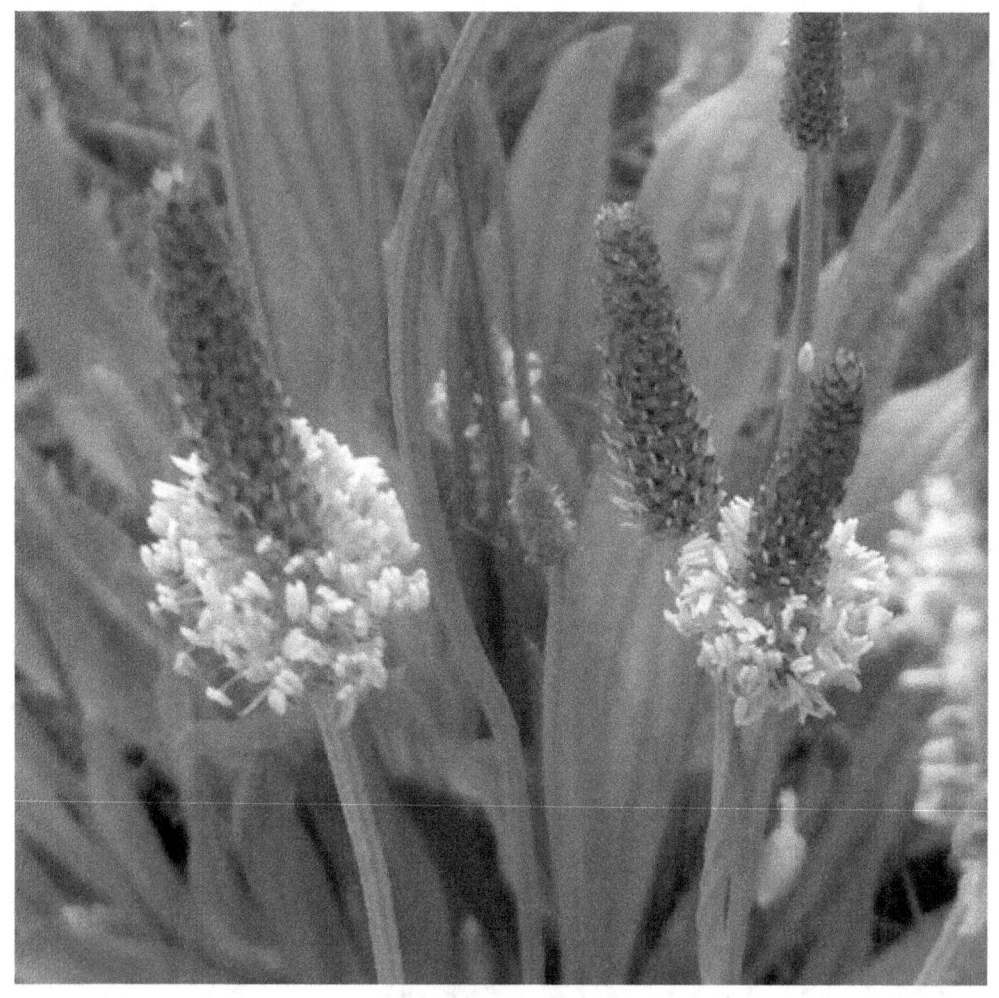

Plantago Lanceolata

Plantain Benefits:

- Respiratory infections.
- Heals cuts
- Treats constipation.
- Relieves boils and acne
- Treats insect bites and stings.
- Soothes irritated eyes.

- Treats burns.
- Relief for coughs and colds..
- Helps eczema and psoriasis.
- Good for the digestion.
- Soothes hemorrhoids.
- Treats mouth ulcers.

All of the above herbs can also be used as an oil or as a poultice. To prepare the Green Salve as a salve take the three equal parts (by weight) of the herbs mentioned and cover them in a pan completely with the olive oil. Simmer on low heat for about 20 to 25 minutes. Then strain out the herbs (after you let it cool for a bit) and keep the oil.

Now place the oil back in the pan and put it back on low heat. Start to add beeswax a little at a time and periodically test the oil in a spoon to see if it turns to a soft salve. You do this by letting the oil in the spoon cool for a minute. If it turns into a soft waxy salve then you should be fine. Please be aware that if you add too much wax then when the salve cools it will become a very hard block and difficult to use. Apply it as often as needed throughout the day for itch relief.

This is **NOT** to be used for fungal type rashes. I will discuss that issue later in this section.

HERBADYNE:

Another formula we have used with great success is a tincture (alcohol based) we call Herbadyne. It's original name was Jethro Kloss herbal liniment. It is considered the herbal sister to Betadine or Iodine. It has been very effective against such issues as poison oak, ivy, sumac as well as against the shingles virus and it's lesions. It is made with Myrrh, Golden seal and cayenne pepper. The beauty of a tincture is it's ability to last long term. I know of someone who likes to collect medieval tinctures. They were created around year 1450. They are still as good to this day as they were made with an alcohol base.

To make this formula;

Ingredients are 2 ounces of powdered Myrrh, one ounce powdered Golden seal, ½ ounce of powdered cayenne and one quart of 100 proof vodka.

Combine all of the herbs and alcohol in a glass jar, cap tightly and keep it in a cool, shaded area for 14 days. Shake at least once each day. Strain it and keep the alcohol in a dark bottle and store in a cool place.

As stated, we have used it very successful for most scrapes and rashes. It can help with fungal rashes as well. We have seen it begin to clear up poison oak as well as shingles within 12 hours. Just apply frequently throughout the day. We use it for all types of scrapes and cuts, to both treat and to prevent infection.

Fungal Type Rashes:

Fungal type rashes include yeast (also seen in diaper rashes) impetigo, and ringworm. Fungal infections are fairly common. Yeasts are botanically related to fungi and can cause skin rashes. These tend to affect folds of skin (like the skin under the breasts or the groin). They look fiery red and have pustules (blisters) around the edges.

Fungal rashes are not commonly acquired from dogs or other animals. They seem to be most easily acquired in gyms, showers, pools, or locker rooms, or from other family members. If a fungus has been repeatedly treated without success, it is worthwhile considering the possibility that it was never really a fungus to start with but rather a form of eczema.

Ringworm, fungal

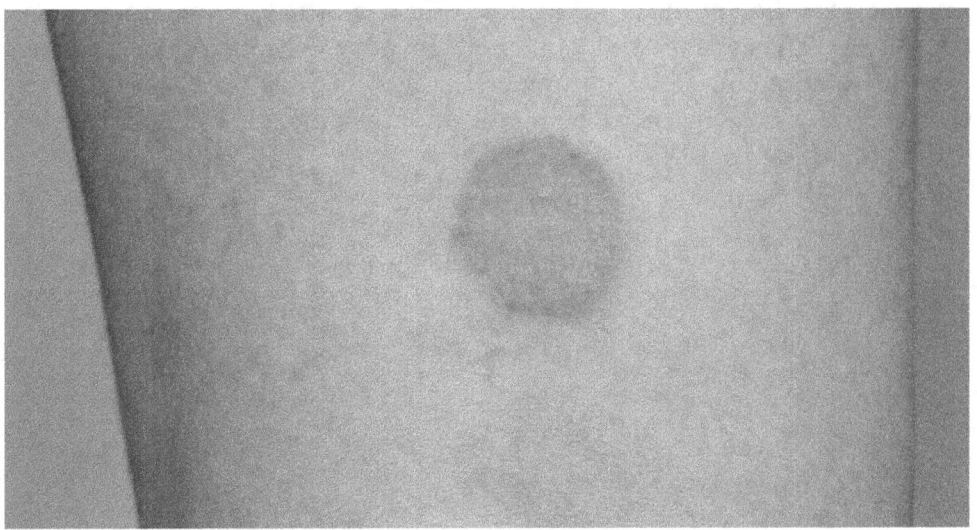

These types of rashes include:

- Most cases of diaper rash
- Ringworm
- Candida rashes
- Tinea
- Athletes foot
- Jock itch

A major cause of these rashes is a weakened immune system.

Treatment here is different since fungal rashes are basically a form of "plant" and we do not want to give it any moisture. There are many wonderful alternative treatments and each rash may require a different protocol.

Treatment #1:

One of the best treatment we have found for stubborn fungal rashes is the use of a solution made from distilled water and Braggs Apple Cider Vinegar.

We usually start off with a 50/50 solution of distilled water and Braggs. Scrub the rash several times a day. It can show a difference within one day. **DO NOT STOP** until the rash is completely gone. If needed, you can do a stronger solution of the Apple cider vinegar but that depends on how sensitive your skin is and how well it tolerates the vinegar.

Treatment #2:

One herb that has been very successful with diaper rash, as well as other fungal types is Black Walnut. We use it in an olive oil and beeswax salve.

Black walnut benefits:

- Supports healthy skin in cases of pimples, skin blemishes, acne breakouts, Psoriasis and eczema.
- It can banish warts.
- Kills parasites.
- Kills fungal infections.
- Improve digestion
- Even found to fight cancer!
- Support heart health.
- Soothes a sore throat.

Not bad, eh? More effective than any pharmaceutical I am aware of. Apply everyday and put a bandage over and change each day. In the case of diaper rash, simply apply several times a day without a bandage. Please be aware that many children and some adults are **VERY** sensitive to the latex and glue in bandages and I have seen cases where the damage from the bandage was worse than the original issue.

7.3 Bites and Stings

With warmer weather comes our neighbors from the forests and fields. Insects and other creatures such as snakes come out to do what comes natural to them but often a torment to the humans. Here we are going to go over some of the things you can do at home to remedy these occurrences.

There are multitudes of different little ones out there who can leave their mark. There are bees, wasps, bed bugs, ticks, mosquitoes, spiders, snakes, etc. Let's look at the symptoms and what we can do for them.

- Bedbugs leave a small bite mark on the skin that is red and itchy or causes a serious allergic reaction.
- Bee stings cause a red skin bump with white around it.
- Flea bites leave an itchy welt on the skin, often on the ankles and legs.
- Mosquitoes leave a raised, itchy pink skin bump or in rare cases a severe allergic reaction.
- Spider bites cause minor symptoms like red skin, swelling, and pain at the site or very serious symptoms that need emergency care.
- Ticks can carry Lyme disease and their bite can leave (only 20% of the time) a rash that looks like an expanding bull's-eye.

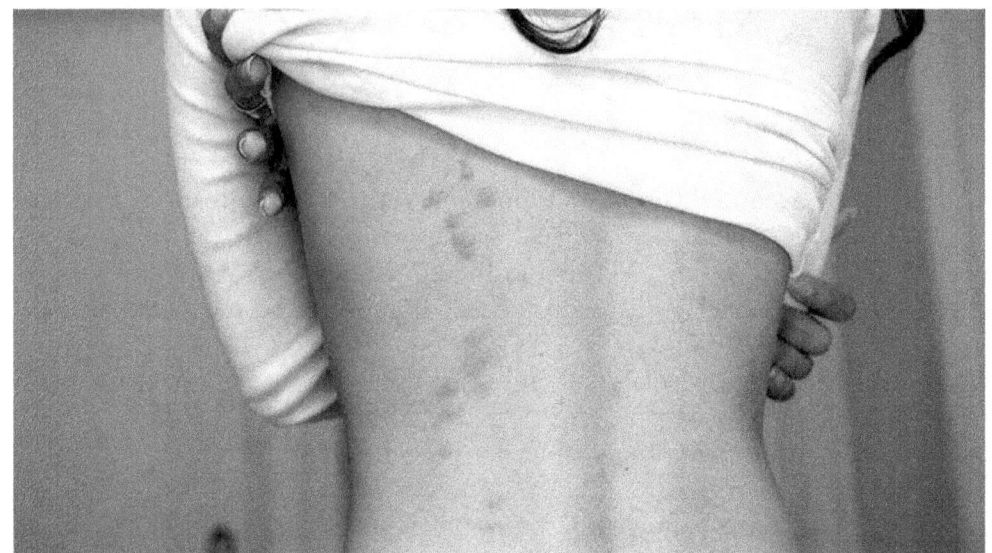
Bed bug bite marks

Usually, the reason bed bug bites become an issue is due to you having an allergic reaction to them. Not everyone has this issue. But if you do, it can be very simple to treat.

First thing of course is to manage the itch. Scratching can lead to greater damage and infection. Here are some simple, at home herbal treatments:

Poke: The skin is an indicator of toxicity in the body. Poke is a good aid for skin problems. It is also good for "the itch" in cases of scabies. Anytime you have skin which doesn't eliminate properly along with vitiated blood, you can well use Poke. It is said to be a great eliminator of toxins out of the system. Usually the glands are not performing properly in these conditions so the herb works on both areas. It is often used in chronic eczema, syphilitic eruptions, psoriasis, varicose veins and leg ulcers.

A mixture of chickweed, olive oil and bees wax makes a great anti-ointment.

Our **Herbadyne** tincture described above works well as it also kills the scabies and bed bugs and relives the itching from them. A solution of distilled water and Braggs Apple Cider Vinegar, 50/50 solution, bathed over the bite can also help relive the itch.

So what do you do if it does becomes infected? The **Green Salve** mentioned earlier works very well for drawing out the poison and the infection. Back many years ago, when I was still early in my lessons on natural first aid, I was bitten by a spider. I thought it would be a great idea to put fresh garlic on the wound. Not a good thing to do. Fresh garlic juice can actually burn the skin. The next day I woke up to a very serious infection and open sore on my hand. Garlic is a wonderful anti-bacterial and natural antibiotic when taken internally or used topically in an olive oil base, but NOT directly on the skin.

I immediately went out and did what I should have done in the first place. I looked for some Plantain growing in the yard. This plant, as shown in the previous section grows all around the world and throughout the United States. Most consider it a weed and that is a shame and a loss. It is wonderful at wound care as it is very efficient at drawing out the infection and sealing the wound quickly.

I made a poultice of the fresh plant that I had gathered. To do this I placed the fresh plants, after I had crushed them and broken up the leaves, into a pan of water. I steeped them at a low temperature for about twenty minutes or so. I then took them out, and after a little cooling so they would not scald, I placed them soaking directly onto the wound. I then wrapped it with a cloth bandage to keep the wet plant material on the wound. I left it on overnight. There are occasions where you will need to change it a couple of times a day.

When I woke the next morning I removed the bandage. I was shocked at the change. Not only was the redness of the infection gone but so was the pus itself. The wound had also closed and was well on it's way to being healed.

SPIDER BITES

Since we're on the subject of spiders, let's talk about treating these dreaded and often scary injuries. There are definitely occasions when you need to seek proper medical care such as in the case of the brown recluse or the black widow and I am not advocating doing this on your own. But ... there are also occasions when you may not have access to a qualified healthcare provider and you need to take the situation into your own hands.

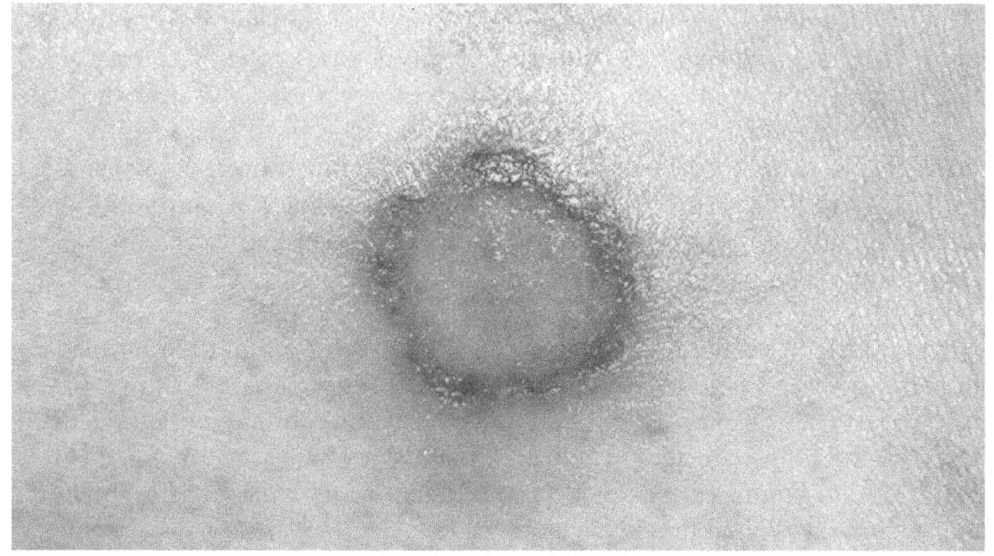

Example of a spider bite

One of the first things you can do is use the above poultice with Plantain. It is amazing at drawing out the poison. I also highly recommend using Poke root in the poultice and orally. You can put a dropper full or more of the Poke root onto the wound before you put the Plantain plant material on top of it. Poke, while it can cause you to throw up, if taken carefully, will not cause it and will help to neutralize the poison internally. At the time of the bite you can take a dropper full every half hour to an hour for at least five hours orally.

As stated earlier, you may need to change the poultice several times during the day to be most effective for drawing out the poison. After about a day you can start using salve like the green salve mentioned earlier. But again, seek medical aid if needed.

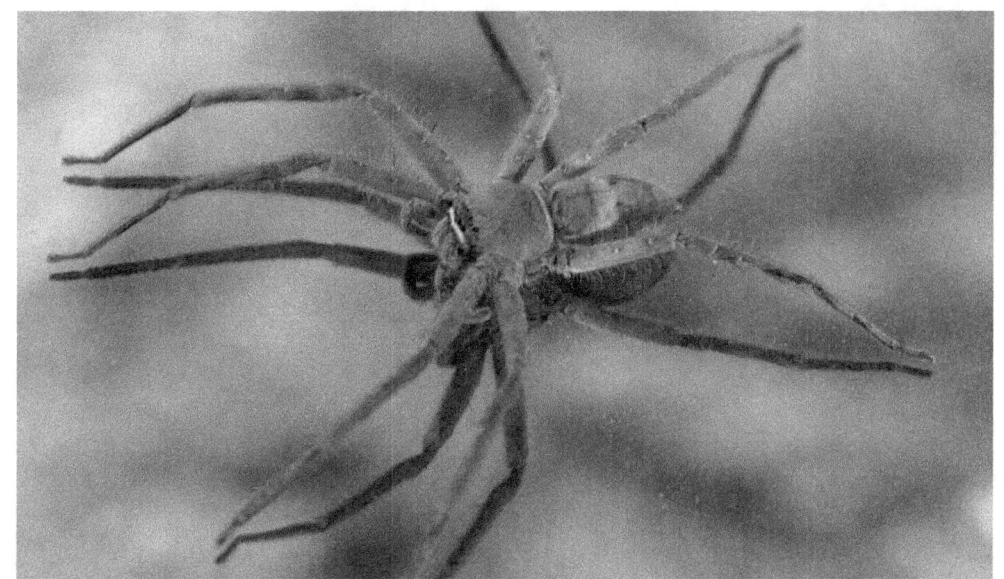
Brown Recluse spider

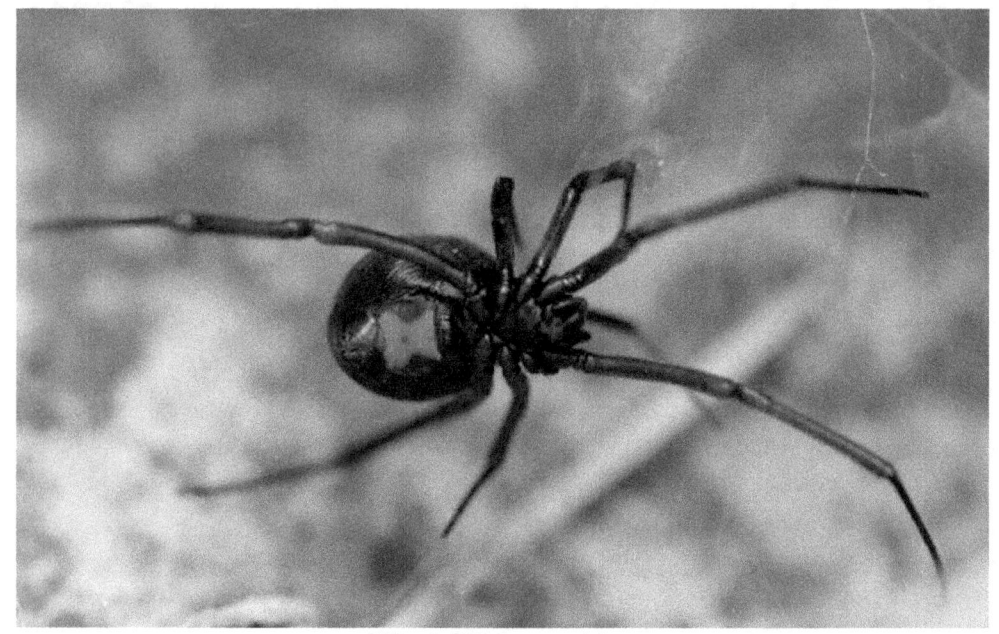

Black Widow spider

A good start is to also avoid being bitten or stung. There are a variety of natural insect repellents. As we go on our outings and picnics this summer, we dread the thought of insects: their stings, bites, annoyances, and the like. We invest in gallons of insect repellents which are expensive and possibly toxic. It is our purpose here to suggest some natural remedies to the problem of being bugged. Some of the simplest insect repellents can be made from our local herbs.

Chamomile and **Yarrow** are two of the best insect repellents in the field. Make a tea of either of these and wash the skin with them and insects will avoid you like the plague. This includes flies, mosquitoes, and their ilk. Because the cosmetic industry uses chaparral as an antiseptic lotion for insect bites, the tea of chaparral may also be tried as a repellent. A member of the family that includes potatoes, cayenne, and eggplant, also includes tobacco, which was used as a successful insect repellent for centuries. In fact, the Indians gave White man tobacco in order to drive them away from the continent. That is why we are taken aback at the reference to Indians smoking a "peace pipe" containing tobacco.

Feverfew: A tincture of the herb, applied locally, is used to relieve pain and swelling caused by bites of insects and vermin. An effective insect repellant is claimed by adding two teaspoonfuls of tincture to one half pint of cold water and then sponging any exposed parts of the body with it.

Chiggers: These are the scourge of the midwest. To repel them, use the aforementioned herbs. To allay the itch produced by their bites, either Chickweed or plantain ointment can be applied. Plantain is an excellent remedy to apply to the site of the bite. It is a blood purifier that will even rally to the occasion of a scorpion bite. It will reduce the red streaks of blood poisoning like no man-made remedy can.

Crushed Onions: Ant bites stop stinging with a poultice of crushed onions.

Pennyroyal: The oil of pennyroyal is a first-rate protection against insect bites (mosquitoes, gnats, and other similar winged pests). It should not be used during pregnancy.

SNAKE BITES:

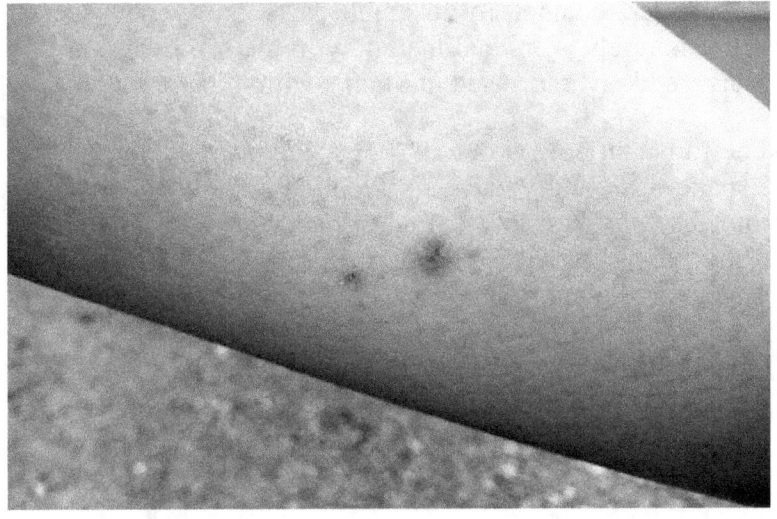

Snake bite

Needless to say, this can often be another occasion when you may want to opt for a qualified healthcare professional. But, as stated, before, that may not be an option. So what are some of the statistics on being bitten by a snake?

As stated by Wikipedia: The United States has about 20 species of venomous snakes, which include 16 species of rattlesnakes, two species of coral snakes, one species of cottonmouth (or water moccasin), and one species of copperhead. At least one species of venomous snake is found in every state except Hawaii and Alaska.

It has been estimated that 7,000–8,000 people per year receive venomous snake bites in the United States, and about five of those people die. Most fatal bites are attributed to the eastern diamondback rattlesnake and the western diamondback rattlesnake. The copperhead accounts for more cases of venomous snake bite than any other North American species; however, its venom is the least toxic, so its bite is seldom fatal.

Venomous snakes are distributed unevenly throughout the United States — the vast majority of snake bites occur in warm weather states. States like Florida and Texas have a wide variety and large population of venomous snakes. Bites from venomous snakes are extremely rare in the states near the Canada–US border. Maine, for example, has only one species (timber rattlesnake); it is rarely seen, and then only in the southern part of the state, but the species is likely extirpated in Maine, with the last sighting in 1901

The good news is that only about 10% of snake bites are fatal. For example, if a rattle snake does bite you, there is only a 15% you even received any venom from the bite and only a 1% chance you will die from it without receiving any care. The very young, elderly and those with a weakened immune system are the most at risk.

HERBAL AIDES:

So, what can be done if you are bitten? Here again, we go back to our champion of the bites and stings ... Plantain.

Plantain: The American Indians used Plantain for a variety of ills. It is said that a South Carolina Indian was given a reward for the information that Plantain was the chief remedy for the cure of rattlesnake bite. Indians are said to have applied a poultice of Plantain for battle bruises and for drawing out snake poisons. The Shoshone Indians made poultices of the whole plant and applied them to the bruises of battles. In some cases, the poultices are combined with the foliage of wild clematis. The Indians of southern Massachusetts applied the leaves both for wounds and for snakebites. The Chippewas used it for inflammation, and as an application to draw out a splinter.

Testimonials:

1. Plantain Leaves and a Sting on the Neck: A 2-year-old was stung on the neck, and the part swelled to enormous size. Again, the remedy was simple, yet wonderfully effective: four plantain leaves were bruised and bound around the neck, and within one hour there was no sign that anything had been wrong with the child.

2. Plantain to the Rescue Again: We have gone on a house call where the hand and arm were swollen up and up the enlarged arm was a red streak with a lump under the arm pit. The individual had blacked out with pain from the wasp sting and swelling. It was early spring and the plantain was not up, so I could not use it fresh. I put plantain ointment, about the size of a dollar, over the sting and within a half an hour the pain was gone. This was in the morning, and they reported back later that the swelling and red streak were gone by afternoon and this boy was out playing ball later that day.

OTHER HERBAL AIDES:

Echinacea: The Omaha Poncas used Echinacea as a basic herb for a variety of ailments. The fresh root was placed on toothaches until the pain subsided. It was used on enlarged glands--like mumps. A smoke fumigant of Echinacea was used to treat headaches, snakebite.

Black Cohosh: The bruised root, applied to the wound, was used by the Indians as an antidote for snakebite, with the juice in small amounts taken internally, apparently by chewing bits of the root.

7.4 Lice

Louse - a general name for various degraded parasitic insects; the true lice that infest mammals belong to the suborder Anoplura Capitus, or head louse; P. Corporis, the body or clothes louse; and Phthirus, or crab louse which lives in the hair upon the pubis, and the eye lashes and eye brows.

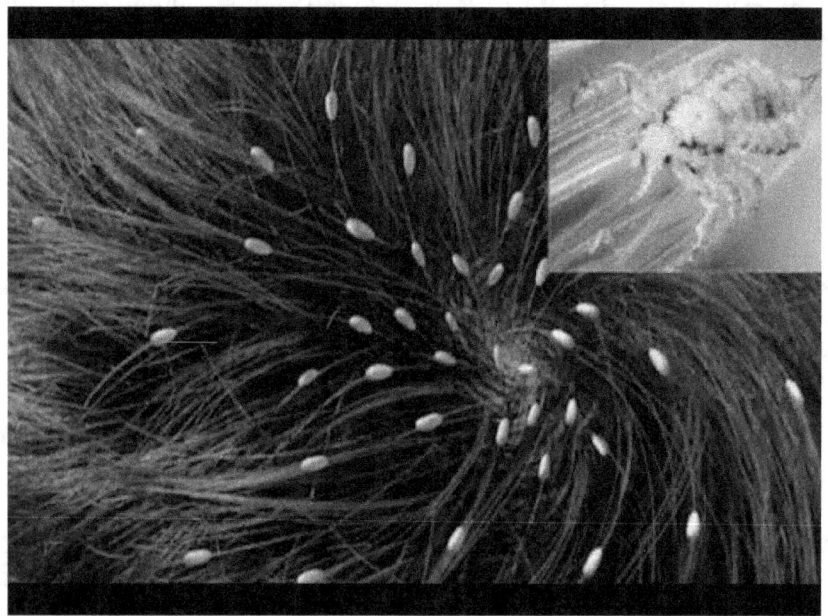

Lice

The causal organisms of typhus fever, relapsing fever, trench fever, and possibly plague are transmitted by the bites of lice. Head lice will never stay around the body that is completely healthy, with no toxins or accumulations of mucus. Lice and all body vermin are scavengers and cannot exist long with clean healthy cells. Keep the bowels clean, stay on a mucusless diet, bathe daily, and lice will not appear.

As recommended by Dr. Christopher: For quick relief (working on the effect) is to bathe the head or body parts covered with lice with straight apple cider vinegar, oil of garlic or walnut (leaf, bark or nut husk) tea. When lice are detected in the family, see that in addition to working on the cause (cleaning the bowel and blood stream) and staying on a mucusless diet, work on the effect itself as suggested here. See that fresh clothes--inner and outer clothing--are changed daily. All of these clothes should be washed with a good biodegradable soap with a cup or more of apple cider vinegar to each washerful of clothes. Change the bed linen each day. Spray the room with tea made of six parts chaparral, three parts black walnut leaf or bark, one part lobelia and to each pint of the spray add some lavender oil or oil of mint to give fragrance.

Another general recommendation by Dr. Christopher included a specific treatment when they are present. Create an infusion of six parts hyssop (Hyssopus officinalis), one part walnut leaves or inner bark (Juglans cinerea), one half part cinnamon bark powder, one half part cloves powder, one half part lobelia, and one half part ginger (Zingiber officinale).

DOSAGE: 1/2 cup (more or less according to age) three times in a day, taken orally. Make fomentation over the head with the same formula, and in other areas infected; covering the fomentation with a plastic or rubber cap at night. Do this six days a week as many weeks as needed to clear up the condition.
Please also remember, a clean house and clean body are not to the liking of our scavenger friends, lice, mites, fleas, etc.

7.5 Warts

As defined by Wikipedia: **Warts** are typically small, rough, hard growths that are similar in color to the rest of the skin. They typically do not result in other symptoms, except when on the bottom of the feet, where they may be painful. While they usually occur on the hands and feet, they can also affect other locations. One or many warts may appear. They are not cancerous.

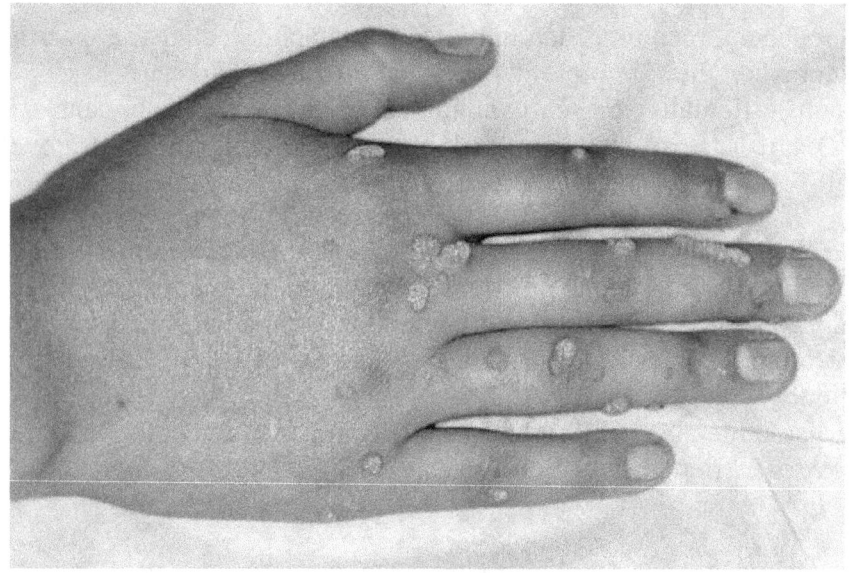

Warts

Warts are caused by infection with a type of human papillomavirus (HPV). Factors that increase the risk include use of public showers, working with meat, eczema and a weak immune system. The virus is believed to enter the body through skin that has been damaged slightly. A number of types exist, including "common warts", plantar warts, "filiform warts", and genital warts. Genital warts are often sexually transmitted

As with most human conditions, warts are usually the result of a nutritional deficiency (most often potassium) and they should be treated internally, as well as externally.

Without treatment, most types of warts resolve in months to years. A number of treatments may speed resolution including salicylic acid applied to the skin and cryotherapy. In those who are otherwise healthy, they do not typically result in significant problems. Treatment of genital warts differs from that of other types.

Warts are very common, with most people being infected at some point in their lives. The estimated current rate of non-genital warts among the general population is 1–13%. They are more common among young people. The estimated rate of genital warts in sexually active women is 12%. Warts have been described at least as far back as 400 BC by Hippocrates

Fortunately, there are a large number of natural cures for warts. As recommended by Dr. Christopher: "The warts, moles and skin blemishes are helped externally and are often cleared up by using the white milk from dandelions and/or from milkweed. Applying castor oil or garlic oil to the area several times a day and taping a piece of gauze soaked with this oil over the wart during the night will aid in clearing the condition. The use of a clove of garlic cut in half (or mashed or grated) and kept over the wart all night until it is gone has aided many."

Black walnut tincture and the following combination tincture have been used with such success that a number of people swear by them. The combination tinctures consists of Blue vervain, Black cohosh, Blue cohosh, Skullcap and Lobelia herbs [Ear and Nerve Tincture] in equal parts, using 90 proof or stronger alcohol as a base.

Potassium Deficiency for Warts and Moles: When cysts or tumors grow in places where they can be seen outside the body, often we react by having them cut out. This defeats healing by working on the effect instead of the cause. You can cut cysts out, tumors off, and burn warts off (which are also a potassium deficiency), or get rid of as many moles as you wish, but unless you go to the cause, they will grow back again, and you may end up with as many or more cysts, tumors, moles as before. Different signs of potassium deficiency will keep popping out on the body because the condition that needs correcting is on the inside. You have to go into the cause, Dr. Christopher always insisted, which is the way we have been eating.

Potassium sources: There are several ways to receive your potassium. Dr. Bernard Jensen sells a potassium broth made from dehydrated vegetables. Dr. Bronner makes a similar, excellent product. You can also make your own potassium broth by simmering equal parts of red potatoes, celery, carrots, onions, and herbs to taste. Raw vegetable and fruit juices also flood the system with potassium.

7.6 Abrasions/bruises

As defined by Wikipedia: An **abrasion** is a partial thickness wound caused by damage to the skin and can be superficial involving only the epidermis to deep, involving the deep dermis. Abrasions usually involve minimal bleeding. Mild abrasions, also known as *grazes* or *scrapes*, do not scar or bleed because the dermis is left intact, but deep abrasions that disrupt the normal dermal structures may lead to the formation of scar tissue. A more traumatic abrasion that removes all layers of skin is called an avulsion.

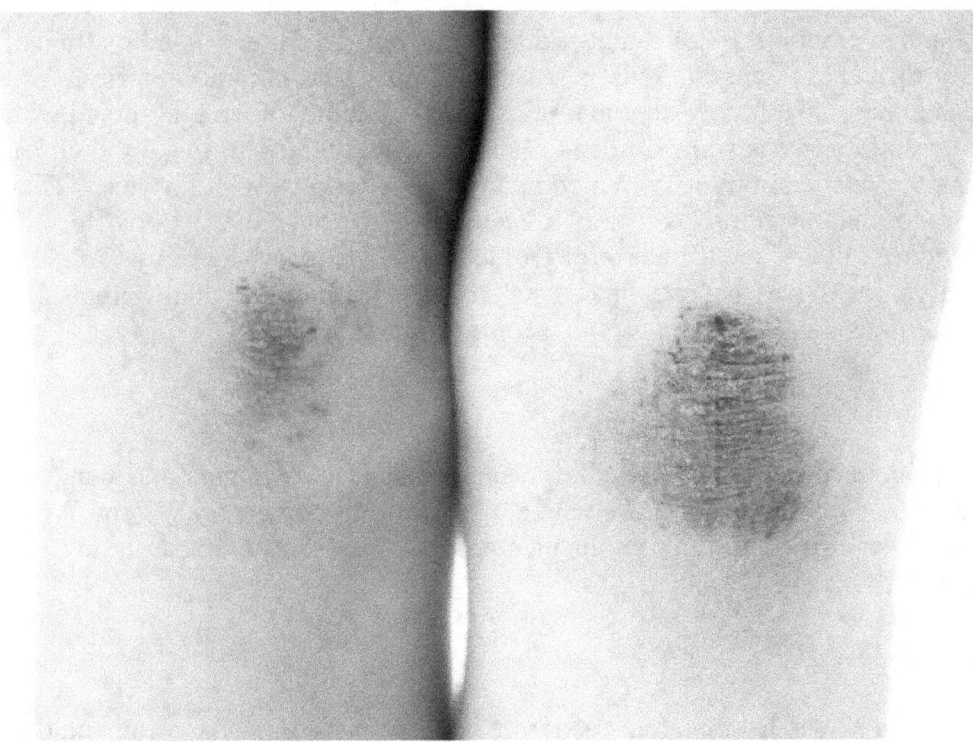

An abrasion

Like much that we have discussed in this chapter, these are usually very simple to treat naturally with little risk of infection.

The first thing I teach my students is to make sure and treat the open scrape with a herbal disinfectant such as Herbadyne. I gave you the instructions on how to make it on page 26. Apply at least once a day, the more the better. It will sting just like Iodine but I have never in over 20 years seen anyone become infected after it's proper use. Once the Herbadyne is applied I then put a healing salve on top of it.

As mentioned before, one of the best aids for scrapes and such is the paste made from Comfrey, raw honey and wheatgerm oil. I described how to make it on page 15. Just apply and cover with a cloth bandage and change at least once a day. It should heal very quickly. You can also use the Green salve mentioned earlier as well. Either works well.

Another wonderful salve that works very well is from a combination of Myrrh and Goldenseal. This is extremely anti-bacterial and anti-viral. You can either make it up with equal parts of Myrrh and Golden seal mixed with olive oil and bees wax, similar to how I discussed how to make the Green salve or you can buy it from a company I have worked with for years. They are located at https://www.rawlife.com/black-herbal-salve/. Look for the product called Country Comfort Goldenseal-Myrrh Herbal Savvy. This is a marvelous salve that we have used on a large number of different skin conditions ranging from a simple scrape to cancer.

BRUISES:

Very common in childhood, they can also appear as bumps and bangs in adulthood, especially in those with a compromised circulatory system. While not necessarily a first aid moment, for some they can be embarrassing and unsightly.

HERBAL AIDS:

Plantain shines here again as a simple cure for bruises. Make a fomentation as described earlier or apply with the Green salve which has Plantain in it.

The Comfrey paste discussed above will also help diminish a bruise quite quickly.

CHAPTER 8

INTERMEDIATE FIRST-AID

Within this chapter I will discuss the next level of emergencies we could face without the help of a qualified health care provider. I will cover how to treat ear infections, eye injuries, minor dental mishaps, allergic reactions, minor bleeding and infections.

As always, please seek help from a qualified health care provider in case of an emergency outside of the scope of your experience.

8.1 Ear Infections

So often they will start with that little itch, a minor annoyance and then can quickly escalate into nights of no sleep and difficulty hearing. We often see it in babies rubbing their ears but children and adults are subject to it's tortures. Sometimes earaches are caused by infection, cold in the head, a blow to the side of the head, and many other causes.

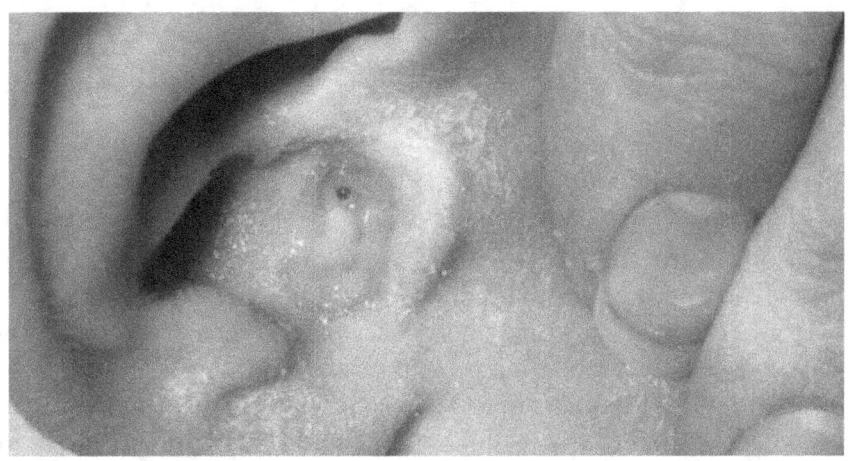

What is an ear infection?

An ear infection is an inflammation of the middle ear, usually caused by bacteria, that occurs when fluid builds up behind the eardrum. Anyone can get an ear infection, but children get them more often than adults. Five out of six children will have at least one ear infection by their third birthday. In fact, ear infections are the most common reason parents bring their child to a doctor. The scientific name for an ear infection is otitis media (OM). Adults can also get ear infections, but they are less common.

The infection usually affects the middle ear and is called otitis media. The tubes inside the ears become clogged with fluid and mucus. This can affect hearing, because sound cannot get through all that fluid.

If your child isn't old enough to say "My ear hurts," here are a few things to look for:

- Tugging at ears
- Crying more than usual
- Fluid draining from the ear
- Trouble sleeping
- Balance difficulties
- Hearing problems

What are the symptoms of an ear infection?

There are three main types of ear infections. Each has a different combination of symptoms.

- **Acute otitis media** (AOM) is the most common ear infection. Parts of the middle ear are infected and swollen and fluid is trapped behind the eardrum. This causes pain in the ear—commonly called an earache. Your child might also have a fever.
- **Otitis media with effusion** (OME) sometimes happens after an ear infection has run its course and fluid stays trapped behind the

eardrum. A child with OME may have no symptoms, but a doctor will be able to see the fluid behind the eardrum with a special instrument.
- **Chronic otitis media with effusion** (COME) happens when fluid remains in the middle ear for a long time or returns over and over again, even though there is no infection. COME makes it harder for children to fight new infections and also can affect their hearing.

In the clinic we have seen wonderful success with just a few simple remedies. Fortunately, nature provides a wonderful medicine cabinet full of natural "antibiotics" and anti-infectives.

HERBAL AIDS:

Garlic: Earache, inflammation of the middle ear, ear disease: Pack a small clove of garlic in gauze and place into the external ear passage; or drop 4-5 drops of Oil of Garlic into the ear channel, cover with flannel, and keep warm.

Mullein: Use warm mullein oil, 2-3 drops in the ear 2-3 times daily. Apple cider vinegar is also a healing agent.

Remember to always treat Both Ears: The simple, old-fashioned aids are sometimes very fast in giving relief. Always treat both ears, even if only one aches.

The lowly **onion** is also a powerful agent in healing. Lightly bake a large onion, cut it in half and while warm (not hot enough to irritate the area), bind one half of the onion over each ear. Bandage in place and hold bandage on with a nightcap, white skullcap, etc., and leave on all night

Dr. Christopher also has an amazing formula as a tincture which we have used very successfully over the years with our patients called the **Ear & Nerve Formula**: Dr. Christopher's Nervous System Formula with Black Cohosh: When this procedure is used as explained here, it can be helpful in promoting an improvement of poor equilibrium, failure of hearing, aiding the motor nerve, etc. With an eye dropper insert into each ear at night four to six drops of oil of garlic and four to six drops of the following herb tincture: blue Cohosh, Black cohosh, Blue vervain, Skullcap, and Lobelia, plugging ears overnight with cotton, six days a week, four to six months, or as needed. On the seventh day, flush ears with a small ear syringe using warm apple cider vinegar and distilled water half and half.

A few testimonials by Dr. Christopher.

1. **Garlic**: When my little girl had an earache I put a piece of fresh garlic in her ear and it was better by morning. The previous alternative was to go to the doctor and pay a lot of money for penicillin.

2. **Super Garlic Immune**: Dr. Christopher's Immune System Support Formula: The Super Garlic Immune formula contains Black Walnut. When Dr. Christopher was lecturing in Snowflake Arizona, he was describing the need for people to be prepared for the coming plagues in the last days.

Someone raised his hand and asked what should be used for the plague. Dr. Christopher, though he was a most noted herbalist, didn't have a ready answer! After a short prayer, he gave the Super Garlic Immune formula to the audience and then just forgot about it. Not long after, people began asking him for the formula again, as those at the Snowflake lecture had made it up and had, had marvelous results; they had cleared up flu, earache, eruptive diseases, car-sickness, and had even saved the life of a poisoned puppy! This Super Garlic Immune remedy is a most valuable combination.

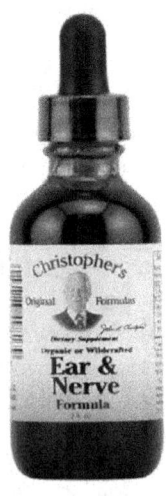

8.2 Dental

Here is a medical issue that can bring a grown man to his knees and not think twice about running to a dentist. There is little that is more painful or life disabling than a dental issue such as tooth infection or mouth sores. You cannot eat and it can even lead to heart issues in the future if not cared for properly. In the more severe cases you will be going to a dentist, but there are many times when it can be cared for successfully at home. Dr. Christopher was very successful with dental issues.

As stated by him: "Tooth problems start several generations back. The weakness of calcium deficiency is passed from parent to child. By following the same parental pattern of "poor food selection," each new crop of babies becomes weaker. "The sins (of omission and of commission) of the parents are passed on to the third and fourth generation." While the baby is being carried in the womb, Mother Nature is interested in that which is being produced more than the one producing. She is continually trying to upgrade humans and animals by drawing on the mother to supply the child. How often do we hear the expression, "Well, I'm carrying another child, that means more varicose veins and loss of more teeth - I don't see why mothers have to suffer this way." Please don't blame the Lord for these conditions, rather blame the use of pastries, soda pop, candy, sugar, ice cream, etc. The sugar leaches the calcium out of the body. Pregnancy is a strain on body calcium, because the mother must have enough calcium in her body for both her and the baby being formed, and later for nursing. If there is not enough calcium for her, because of this leaching process by the sugar (of past and present), the fetus draws on the mother's body. The calcium it now takes is from the bones, muscles, and the teeth, etc. Sometimes so much is taken from the mother that she will, after a number of babies, have bone and muscle problems from a great lack of calcium.

When a child is being formed and there is not enough calcium being supplied to the fetus, the jaw of the child will not form fully. It will be narrow instead of broad. When it is time for the child to cut teeth, they cannot come in "Straight" because of a crowded jaw space. So, naturally, they will come in crooked. Later as there is not enough room for the wisdom teeth, they must often be extracted before coming through. When the day comes that the jaw is adequately large and well-shaped to accommodate all thirty-two teeth without crowding them to crookedness, and the wisdom teeth can remain until old age (and in comfort), it will mean we humans have "gained enough wisdom" to keep them!

The basic cause of calcium loss, of course, as mentioned, is leaching out the calcium with sugars and a toxic body condition. Nearly all tooth decay comes from the blood stream, saliva, and the inside of the teeth, not only from the external surface. The teeth deteriorate but it is from the toxic blood stream and the enamel-destroying toxic saliva which is a result of an impure (toxic) blood stream. If a child has good wholesome food and has been given a "good solid start in life" with a full healthy set of teeth and jaws, he can go through life without tooth problems. The condition of perfect teeth is, of course, dependent upon a continual use of wholesome and proper foods."

One way to accomplish this level of calcium is to use a formula Dr. Christopher's created called **Calc-Tea**. Calc-Tea is made of Horsetail grass, Oat straw, Comfrey leaves and Lobelia. Horsetail grass and Oat straw are high in silica. Calcium can't be used in the body without the presence of Silica. The other Herbs support the function of the silica herbs in helping the body assimilate calcium.

> The formula is as follows:
> 6 parts Horsetail grass (Equisetum hyemale)
> 3 parts Oat straw (Avena sativa)
> 4 parts Comfrey root (Symphytum officinale)
> 1 part Lobelia (Lobelia inflata)

In this case a part is measured in weight, such as ounces. It can taken as a tea with one teaspoon to a cup of water or a tablespoon to a pint. It can also be taken in capsules.

The following testimonials attest to it's efficiency:

1. **Tooth Grows Back**: My oldest daughter age 13 now, had a dental cavity at age 7 (the only dental cavity among our six children). We had the cavity drilled out and a filling put in by our local dentist. Two years later, the filling

came out and a hole was left in her tooth. Nothing more was done about it except the herbal calcium formula that you recommend in your book, School of Natural Healing, made up of: Comfrey, horsetail, Oatstraw, and Lobelia. This combination of herbs has been used very consistently by the entire family over the last two years. We have recently discovered that the hole where the filling was is now completely grown over and is absolutely unnoticeable even under close inspection.

2. **Insomnia Cured**: I have found great relief by taking Dr. Christopher's calcium formula and thyroid formula through the night which was recommended in his "How Important is Calcium" newsletter. I have recommended this treatment to others and to my mother and they all have found it helps their insomnia also. -A.R., Williston, ND.

Sometimes the best defense is a good offense, preventative care. Dr. Christopher stated: "**Children need calcium if bones and teeth are to grow strong and well-formed. Adults need an adequate amount of calcium every day. During periods of pregnancy and lactation, women require much more calcium than normally, as they must also furnish extra calcium for the baby.** "

Another wonderful formula is Dr. Christopher's Herbal Tooth Powder. It can be purchased online or you can make it yourself. It is very easy to make and it is used instead of tooth paste for regularly brushing of your teeth. It is all I have used for years, brushing daily. The formula is as follows:

3 part Oak bark (Quercus alba)
6 parts Comfrey root (Symphytum officinale)
3 parts Horsetail grass (Equisetum hymale)
1 part Lobelia (Lobelia inflata)
1 part Cloves (Syzgyium aromaticum)
3 parts Peppermint (Mnetha piperita)

A nice testimonial for the above tooth powder formula: **No Root Canal**: After breaking a tooth from biting my fingernails, I had to have a crown put on one of my bottom front teeth. This tooth aches all the time. Sometimes it's from the weather, sometimes from eating something, and sometimes from headaches. My tooth was so sensitive I couldn't eat corn on the cob!

When I complained about the pain, my dentist told me that if it keeps bothering me we might have to do a root canal. I started using Dr. Christopher's Herbal Tooth Powder to brush my teeth once or twice a week. As long as I remember to brush with the tooth powder, my tooth doesn't hurt. Whenever I forget to use it, my tooth starts to hurt again. I love the tooth powder, because it helped me avoid a root canal.

HERBAL AIDS:

For tooth pain use Clove oil or Plantain powder on the tooth at the roots.

An excellent treatment with a great history for gum disease and even cavities and blackened teeth uses the above tooth powder along with a Black walnut tincture. Each day, three times a day, brush your teeth with the above tooth powder. When you have finished brushing and have spit out the water now mix in a quarter cup of water with two dropper fulls of the Black walnut tincture. Swish this in your mouth for at least a minute and then swallow it. Do this at this dosage and rate for two weeks. If the gums are improving and the pain is gone you can drop the dosage to one dropper full a day.

I have also seen wonderful success with olive oil pulling. I have heard of others using coconut oil but I believe olive oil is more effective. We use this to aid in drawing out the infection from the teeth and gums. Swish it in your mouth at least three times a day during a serious infection. Hold it in the mouth for at least 10 minutes and then spit it out.

You can also use castor oil packs over an abscess in cases of severe infections or cysts caused by the infections. To do this soak a white cotton cloth in castor oil and place it over the cheek's skin nearest the infection or tooth pain. Now cover the cloth with a saran wrap and then place a towel over the wrap. Next, place a heating pad over the towel Do this as many times a day as you can, at least twice a day. I have seen serious cysts and infection begin to drain in just a couple of days. It may take weeks for the cyst to completely disappear.

8.3 Infections

Hospital-acquired infections with *Staphylococcus aureus*, especially methicillin-resistant *S. aureus* (MRSA) infections, are a major cause of illness and death and impose serious economic costs on patients and hospitals. Nosocomial (hospital acquired infection) bloodstream infections are a leading cause of death in the United States. If we assume a nosocomial infection rate of 5%, of which 10% are bloodstream infections, and an attributable mortality rate of 15%, bloodstream infections would represent the eighth leading cause of death in the United States.

Among the most common types of these infections include MRSA, septicemia and influenza and pneumonia. Infections can be either or both of a bacterial or viral nature. Unfortunately, as the rate in increase of MRSA proves, the bacteria soldiers are winning battle as they become more and more resistant to antibiotics.

The Threat of Antibiotic Resistance

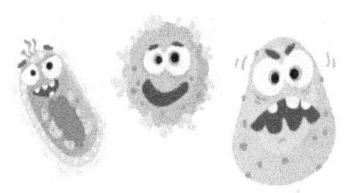

Increase in antibiotic resistance means that the effectiveness of antibiotics used to treat infections is diminished or non-existent.

"The use of antibiotics is the single most important factor leading to antibiotic resistance around the world."

2 Million the number of people in the US that acquire serious antibiotic-resistant infections each year

23,000 the number of people in the US that die as a direct result of antibiotic resistant infections each year

250,000 the number of people in the US that require hospital care for Clostridium difficil *(C. difficile: a unique bacterial infection directly related to antibiotic use and resistance)* infections each year

14,000 the number of people in the US that die from C. difficil infections each year

One of the most commonly prescribed drugs in the United States are antibiotics. According to the CDC:

- 50% of prescribed antibiotics are not needed or are not optimally effective as prescribed.
- 1 out 5 emergency visits are for adverse drug events involving antibiotics.
- $35 billion a year lost to productivity because of antibiotic usage.
- $20 billion estimated yearly excess in direct healthcare costs in part due to prolonged and/or costlier treatments.
- Individuals with an already compromised immune system are made worse by the use of antibiotics.
- At least 70% of Americans have a candida overgrowth due to the use of antibiotics, thereby compromising their immune systems further.

So, what can we do when we are threatened with an infection when going to the hospital has become such a possibly risky trip? The plant kingdom has a wide variety of medicines used successfully throughout history.

HERBAL AIDS:

By far, the best natural antibiotic or anti-infective we have used is hands down, the Stinking Rose, also known as the simple **Garlic**. It is a medical fact that three to five cloves of garlic is the equivalent in efficacy to an adult dose of penicillin, without destroying your gut micro-flora.

Garlic can be used in many ways but it CANNOT be cooked if you want any medicinal value out of it. It has approximately 35 sulfur compounds in it and this makes it such an effective antibiotic and the good news is that even If you are allergic to sulfur types of antibiotics, this one will not hurt you. But this is the reason it cannot be cooked as the compounds are destroyed with heat.

It can be dried and used in capsules. It can also be used in oils. A garlic oil compound is very effective for ear infections and such. To make a garlic oil simply chop up some garlic and put into a bottle and cover completely with olive oil. Shake for three days and then filter out the garlic pieces. That's it. Use the oil as needed.

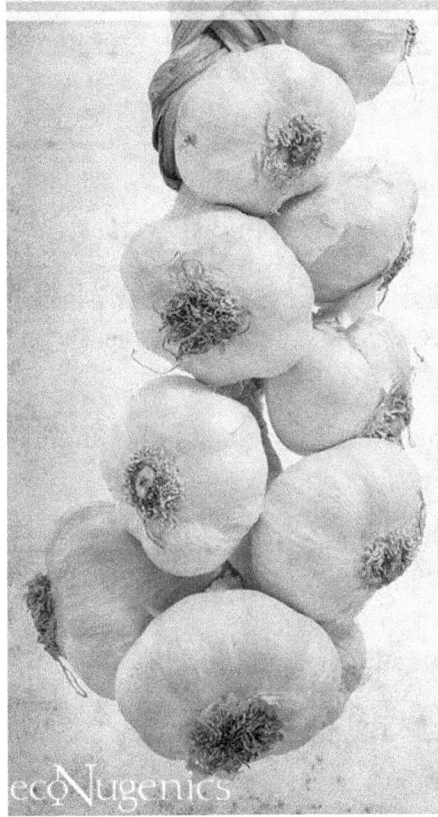

Health Benefits of Garlic

- Boosts Immune System
- Treats Athlete's Food
- Stops Toothaches
- Curbs Cold + Flu Effects
- Lowers Cholesterol
- Treat Insect Bites
- Promote Heart Health
- Clears Nasal Congestion
- Heal Cold Sores
- Kills Parasites
- Lowers Blood Pressure
- Repel Mosquitoes
- Prevent Blood Clots
- Aid Poor Digestion

Another great way to use garlic is as a paste. Please keep in mind that fresh garlic juice can actually burn the skin and this is why it needs to be in an oil or some other kind of salve or paste.

To make as a paste chop up several cloves of garlic and mix with petroleum jelly. This is the only time you will see me recommended this medium but it is basically inert and will hold the garlic while protecting the skin. If someone is ill with an infection or a cold or the flu you can make this paste and place on the bottoms of their bare feet. Cover with a cloth bandage and then their socks. Let them wear it all night. It is interesting to note how quickly garlic can pass into the system. You can place this paste on the feet and in a very short time you will be able to smell it on their breath.

Please remember, the fresher the garlic, the better.
As capsules take 3 or more capsules five times a day internally during an illness or infection.

OTHER HERBAL AIDS:

There are a number of herbs that also work very well for infections.

Onion poultice: This is an old but tried and true practice that has worked wonderfully for respiratory issues such as colds, the flu, bronchitis and even pneumonia. It involves the little cousin to garlic … the onion.

To make the poultice, take a white or yellow onion and chop up thoroughly. Place in the oven at about 250 to 300 degrees for about twenty minutes. You will know when it is done as the pieces are just starting to get "slimy". Now take them out and let them cool enough where they will not damage the skin and place over the chest while the patient is lying down. If this is for a baby then please make sure to rub some olive oil on the skin first to protect it as they are more sensitive than older children or adults.

Now cover the onions with a towel and then a heating pad. Keep on for at least a half an hour. Do this several times a day.

Onion cough syrup: You can also make the onions into an excellent cough syrup. Take a white or yellow onion and chop up and place into a sauce pan. Cover with raw honey and simmer over low heat for about 25 to 30 minutes. Strain and use the honey as a teaspoon to a tablespoon as needed for coughs.

Golden seal is a wonderful anti-viral. For colds and the flu, use three capsules five times a day until the patient is cured.

Echinacea – This herb works wonderfully as it fools the body into believing it was poisoned (though it was not). It causes the immune system to go into high gear. The problem is that after about five days the body realizes it is not being poisoned and will stop working. Take a break for a few days and start back up and the body will have forgotten and will ramp the immune system back up. Take two to three capsules five times a day during an infection or illness. This herb also works very well with Goldenseal.

Coconut oil is very effective when used topically on MRSA skin infections.

Cats Claw – This is an amazing herb for fighting bacteria, second to garlic. I use it when treating Lyme disease and it is very effective in killing the bacteria. Take two capsules five times a day during an illness.

For wound and skin infections please remember to use the **Herbadyne** mentioned in a previous section. Apply topically several times a day during the active part of the infection.

Another formula that has worked very well in the field is Dr. Christopher's **Infection Formula**. I have used it successfully for parasites, bacterial and viral infection and mold type illnesses.

The formula is as follows:

INFECTION FORMULA:

4 parts Plantain (Plantago major)
4 parts Black walnut (Juglans nigra)
4 parts Goldenseal root (Hydransis Canadensis)
2 parts Bugle weed (Lycopus virginicus)
1 part Marshmallow root (Althaea officinalis)
1 part Lobelia (Lobelia inflata)

All parts are measured in weight, for example one part equals one ounce.

During an infection, cold, the flu, etc., you take three capsules five times a day or if it is very serious you can use three to five capsules every hour until the patient improves and then you can drop the dosage to five times a day.

8.4 Allergic reactions

Food allergies are a growing epidemic in the United States with a diagnosis of anaphylactic food reactions increasing by 377 percent from 2007 to 2016. Peanuts are at the top with eggs and sea food coming in second and third. As the diet and quality of food in this nation continues to degrade these types of issues are becoming more common place in American households. The reactions can appear very mild from a simple case of hives and watery eyes and sniffles to a life threatening condition requiring immediate medical intervention, anaphylactic shock.

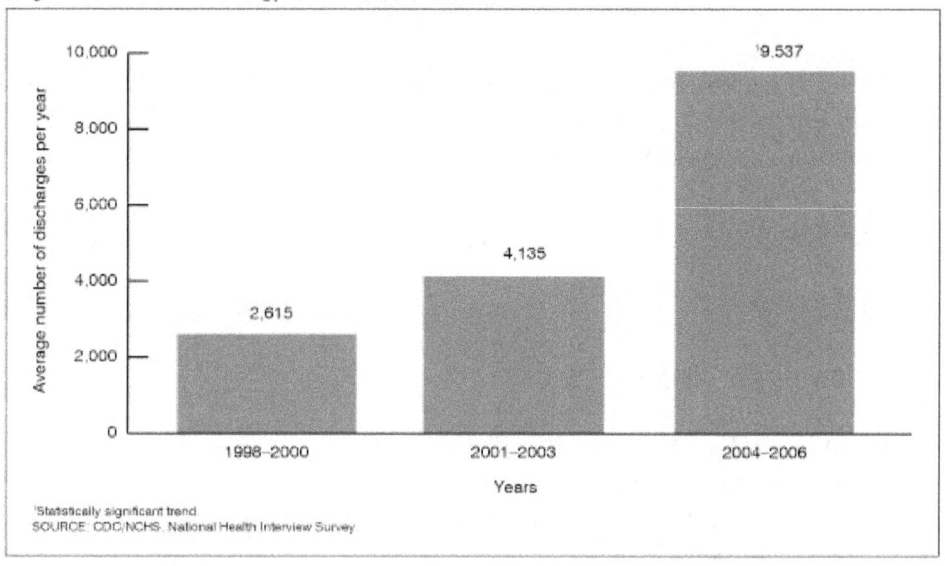

Figure 4. Average number of hospital discharges per year among children under age 18 years with any diagnosis related to food allergy: United States, 1998-2006

According to JAMA, the Journal for the American Medical Association: **The overall economic cost of food allergy was estimated at $24.8 (95% CI, $20.6-$29.4) billion annually ($4184 per year per child). Direct medical** costs were $4.3 (95% CI, $2.8-$6.3) billion annually, including clinician visits, emergency department visits, and hospitalizations. Costs borne by the family totaled $20.5 billion annually, including lost labor productivity, out-of-pocket, and opportunity costs. Lost labor productivity costs totaled $0.77 (95% CI, $0.53-$1.0) billion annually, accounting for caregiver time off work for medical visits. Out-of-pocket costs were $5.5 (95% CI, $4.7-$6.4) billion annually, with 31% stemming from the cost of special foods. Opportunity costs totaled $14.2 (95% CI, $10.5-$18.4) billion annually, relating to a caregiver needing to leave or change jobs.

The current standard treatments today utilizes a series of drugs aimed at suppressing the immune system. These include antihistamines and steroids. For severe allergic reactions the EpiPen is the choice for many. Unfortunately, it's cost has more the quadrupled n the last few years putting it outside of most patient's budgets when they have no insurance.

In this section I will go over a wide range of holistic, herbal medications you can do at home for treating anything from the mild watery eyes to the more severe anaphylactic shock. Always remember to seek a qualified healthcare provider in cases of emergency.

HERBAL AIDS:

Stinging Nettle: This wonderful little plant actually has very similar properties to Benadryl. It acts as an antihistamine, relieving the mild allergic reaction such as hive, watery eyes and sniffles without making you sleepy like Benadryl. We use it as an alcohol based tincture. During a mild allergic event such as seasonal allergies, we usually recommend two dropper fulls three times a day. You can also use it as needed and so you can use it throughout the day during a more severe hay fever attack, for example. It is non-toxic and therefore you will not overdose on it.

Immucalm: This formula was created by Dr. Christopher for calming the immune system while still allowing it to be strong. It is NOT an immune-suppressant and therefore will not leave you open to other infections, such as some of the other drugs can do. It is made from two herbs; Astragalus and

Marshmallow root. It can be purchased online or you can make it yourself at home. It also comes in a gentle glycerin based liquid formula for children.

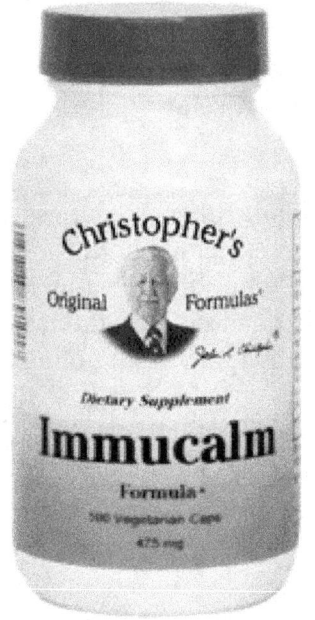 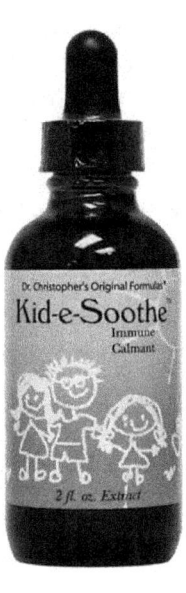

It is very simple to make it yourself. It is equal parts Astragalus and Marshmallow root. This has been used successfully with such issues as hayfever, allergy related asthma, Rheumatoid Arthritis, any auto-immune disease, and any type of hyper-immune disorder.

The above two formulas, Kid-e-Soothe and Stinging Nettle also can play an important part in dealing with anaphylactic shock where an EpiPen is not available. This happened once with a patient who could not afford to pay for the new costs of EpiPens and asked for a natural alternative. I informed her that such an issue is a medical emergency and she needed to be careful about her medical choices. She went ahead and requested the protocol.

This protocol requires having a full and sealed bottle of each of the two medications, Kid-e-Soothe and Stinging Nettle. She was to keep both with her at all times, just like she would with an EpiPen. She was very allergic to insect stings and bites such as a bee and had a history of life threatening reactions. If she were stung or bitten she was to IMMEDIATELY open both bottles and drink them completely as quickly as she could.

Well, it happened. She and a friend were sitting at poolside one day and she suddenly felt the bite on the top of her head. Her friend had been taught what to do and immediately got her friend's purse and cracked open both bottles and had her drink them immediately. She did so and they waited. Nothing happened.

After a few minutes her friend told her she would be in the house washing the dishes but would be watching from the kitchen window. The patient told her she felt fine and to go ahead. After about 20 minutes her friend noted that she seemed to be slumping somewhat in the poolside chair. She ran out to see if she was alright.

The patient, not used to alcohol from the Stinging Nettle, informed her friend she was feeling great but was a bit looped. All was well and she immediately purchased another set of the herbal medications.

OTHER USEFUL AIDS FOR ALLERGIES:

Apple cider Vinegar: Braggs Apple Cider Vinegar is supposed to work well with allergies due to it's ability to cut mucous production and cleanse the lymphatic system. During allergy season just mix a tablespoon or two in a glass of distilled water and drink three times a day.

Neti Pot: For those familiar with it, it is simply a spouted container, similar to a little teapot. You fill it with distilled water and a quarter teaspoon of salt. You use this to rinse out your sinus cavity. Use a pre-made saline rinse or make your own by dissolving 1/4 teaspoon of Himalayan or just plain sea salt in a quart of boiled distilled water. Cool completely. Put in the Neti Pot and pour through one nostril and let it drain out the other. Make sure to do both nostrils.

Raw Local Honey: Raw, local honey from a compassionate bee keeper works very well as it contains pollen from your area. Taking a tablespoon a day all year is like giving yourself a gentle vaccine. The theory is that it gradually and safely builds up an immunity to the pollen and you experience little to no seasonal allergy issues after.

Mullein and Lobelia Tincture: Sometimes during an allergy attack, breathing may become difficult. In lieu of having a rescue inhaler we like to use what was very common among the Native Americans. This utilized the herb called Mullein, a very common plant in the United States. It was well known by them to use it during an asthmatic attack. They would breath in the smoke of the leaves and the attack would stop immediately.

We make it into a tincture of 3 parts Mullein and 1 part Lobelia. We instruct our patients to use a dropper full on the tongue as needed to stop the asthma attack.

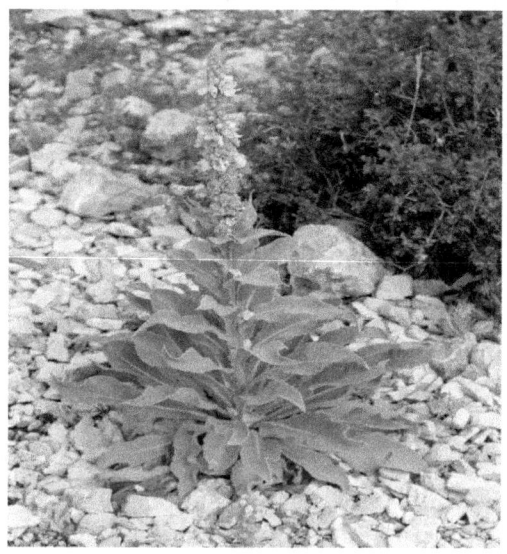

Mullein

Gut Health: As described in my book *A Complete Body Repair, Healing Candida, Parasites and Heavy Metal Toxicity Naturally*, I discuss the importance of a healthy micro-flora colony in the gut. This is 70 to 80% of your immune system and this is a leading cause of allergies as an unhealthy environment can lead to "Leaky Gut Syndrome". I have seen MANY patients lose their allergies when the gut health was restored to a normal condition. I myself used to be very allergic to Poison Oak but no longer experience it once I healed my intestinal environment.

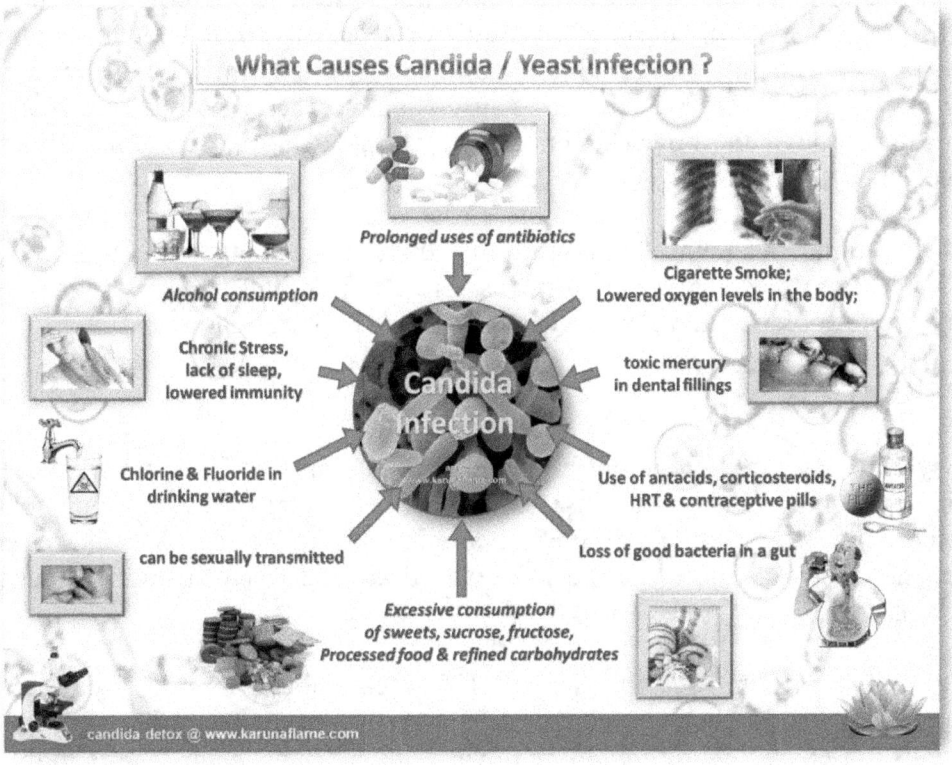

8.5 Bleeding - Minor

One of the most frightening things you can experience at home is an accident with resulting bleeding. As defined by The School of Natural Healing: The escaping of blood internally or externally. Blood coughed from the lungs is generally of a bright red color and is usually mixed with sputum. The problem is often preceded by nausea and stomach disorder with blood passing through the bowels. Simple enough. What do we do about minor events?

This section deals mainly with minor bleeding issues along the lines of cuts, scrapes, nose bleeds and mouth issues. Chapter four will focus more on the very serious bleeding problems, external, internal, during labor and such.

HERBAL AIDS:

Cayenne: By far, I know of NO better styptic than the sizzling cayenne. I have seen miracles with the use of this herb. Dr. Christopher would often remark how you could count to 60 after using this herb and you would often see the bleeding stopped before you reached the end. I have personally seen this happen.

Cayenne is known as a rubefacient. This means that where ever cayenne touches it brings blood to that area. While there are many benefits this brings, for example, bringing more oxygen and nutrients, what we see in this case is an equalization of blood pressure. It simply pulls the pressure off of the wound and slows or stops the bleeding.

In the case of an open wound or nose bleed, simply put a few drops of cayenne tincture on your tongue. You can also use pure cayenne powder as it will work as well. If you are brave, you can also put a small amount of the cayenne into the wound. Yes, it will be very hot but it can stop the bleeding very quickly. Once done, simply count to 60 and watch the results.

My wife is a wonderful example of this. On two separate instances, within a week of each other, provided wonderful proof to cayenne's effectiveness. The first incident involved a mandolin while slicing up zucchini for me. She was slicing the zucchini and grew impatient and removed the blade guard. It was the next slice that removed a small portion of her thumb. Blood began to spurt out of the wound with each heartbeat. Fortunately, she had some holistic first aid training prior to this and immediately grabbed the cayenne tincture we keep on hand for just such emergencies.

She immediately poured some of the cayenne tincture on the counter and rubbed her open wound in it! Needless to say, it was quite hot and painful. The good news is that cayenne causes zero tissue damage, even if it feels as though it is. She also squirted a dropper full in her mouth and then began to count. By the time she hit sixty there was barely an ooze from her open cut.

Well, another incident occurred about a week later. She had finished washing the dishes and they were drying in the dish drainer. When it came to time to put them away, she reached and grabbed a handful of silverware to put in the draw right next to her. In the middle of the handful was a knife pointing down. She relaxed her grip slightly and down went the knife, straight into the top of her foot. She looked down to see a knife standing straight up, embedded in the top of her foot. She is a tough Alabama, Cherokee woman and she knew what to do. She simply reached down and pulled out the knife. Of course, out came the blood. Fortunately, she still had the bottle of cayenne tincture on the counter. She chose this time to not put it straight into the wound but squirted a dropper full into her mouth. Again, she counted. After sixty seconds, the bleeding had completely stopped. A wonderful miracle cayenne is for any home first-aid kit.

HOW TO MAKE CAYENNE TINCTURE:

Making cayenne tincture is a simple process, and the only drawback to making your own is the time spent waiting for the tincture to be ready to use. Cayenne tincture can be made from dried cayenne peppers or cayenne pepper powder.

Pack a 1-quart jar tightly with cayenne peppers. If using whole peppers, make sure to chop them thoroughly to increase surface exposure to the alcohol. If using cayenne pepper powder, fill the jar half-full.

Fill the jar with vodka to within a half-inch of the jar's top. Use apple cider vinegar or glycerin if you don't want to use alcohol.

Place the lid on the jar and tighten.

Store in a cool, dark place for two weeks, making sure to walk by at least once a day and shake vigorously.

Drain the tincture though cheesecloth to remove the peppers from the liquid.

Pour the strained tincture into smaller, colored bottles and cap. Be sure to label the bottles. The tincture will keep indefinitely in a cool area.

Dr. Christopher had wonderful advice for those who suffer with chronic nosebleeds:

Nosebleeds: Unless it is from injury, nosebleed results from a calcium deficiency. It is caused by the rupture of a small vessel in the nose due to pressure in the head. There are many causes for nosebleeds, but the weakness stems from calcium deficiency. Of course, it does not matter how much calcium is in the body if one is hit in the nose with a good blow; bleeding will start. A teaspoon of cayenne in a cup of water (hot preferred) taken internally will stop most nosebleeds quickly. In an emergency such as this we use cayenne. As mentioned a teaspoon of cayenne pepper in a glass of water and drunk right down will stop a nosebleed in nearly every instance, by the time you can count to ten. This is not a miracle; it is the principle of the cell stimulant cayenne traveling through the entire blood stream and regulating the pressure so the pressure of the flow is the same in the feet as in the head or any other part of the body. This takes the heavy pressure off the hemorrhaging area and allowing a quick coagulation. One of our very finest herbal foods is our calcium formula [Herbal Calcium Formula] of four parts Comfrey root, six parts horsetail grass, three parts oat straw and one part Lobelia. Make this into a tea, using a cup (one teaspoon of combined herbs to cup of distilled water) morning and one evening or two or three capsules or tablets two or three times in a day.

Stinging Nettle: In Russia, it is used as a valued antiseptic and astringent. The pulverized dry herb is sniffed to stop nose bleeding.

OTHER HERBAL AIDS:

Shepard's Purse: What a gentle little herb shaped like a heart. There is an ancient theory called the Doctrine of Signatures where it states that plants of a particular shape heals in the body similar. I can see that with this little herb with it's shape and the circulatory system.

As stated by Dr. Christopher: "Most herbalists agree on most of the medicinal qualities of Shepherd's Purse, they being astringent, styptic, diuretic, anti-scorbutic, vasoconstrictor and blood coagulant, which therefore makes it anti-hemorrhagic (or hemostatic). Additionally, Kloss listed it as having detergent and vulnerary qualities.

Grieve said it was anti-diarrheal, Duke mentioned its antioxidant qualities and Schwartz claimed it to be anti-inflammatory. Moore got more specific, mentioning that Shepherd's Purse uses were: "Urinary tract astringent, uric acid diuretic for hyperuricemia; hemostatic for hematuria, excess menses, and so forth; and an oxytocin agonist for postpartum bleeding or difficult placenta delivery."

DOSAGE: For bleeding issues take a teaspoon of the tincture every few minutes or a half a cup every ten minutes until bleeding stops.

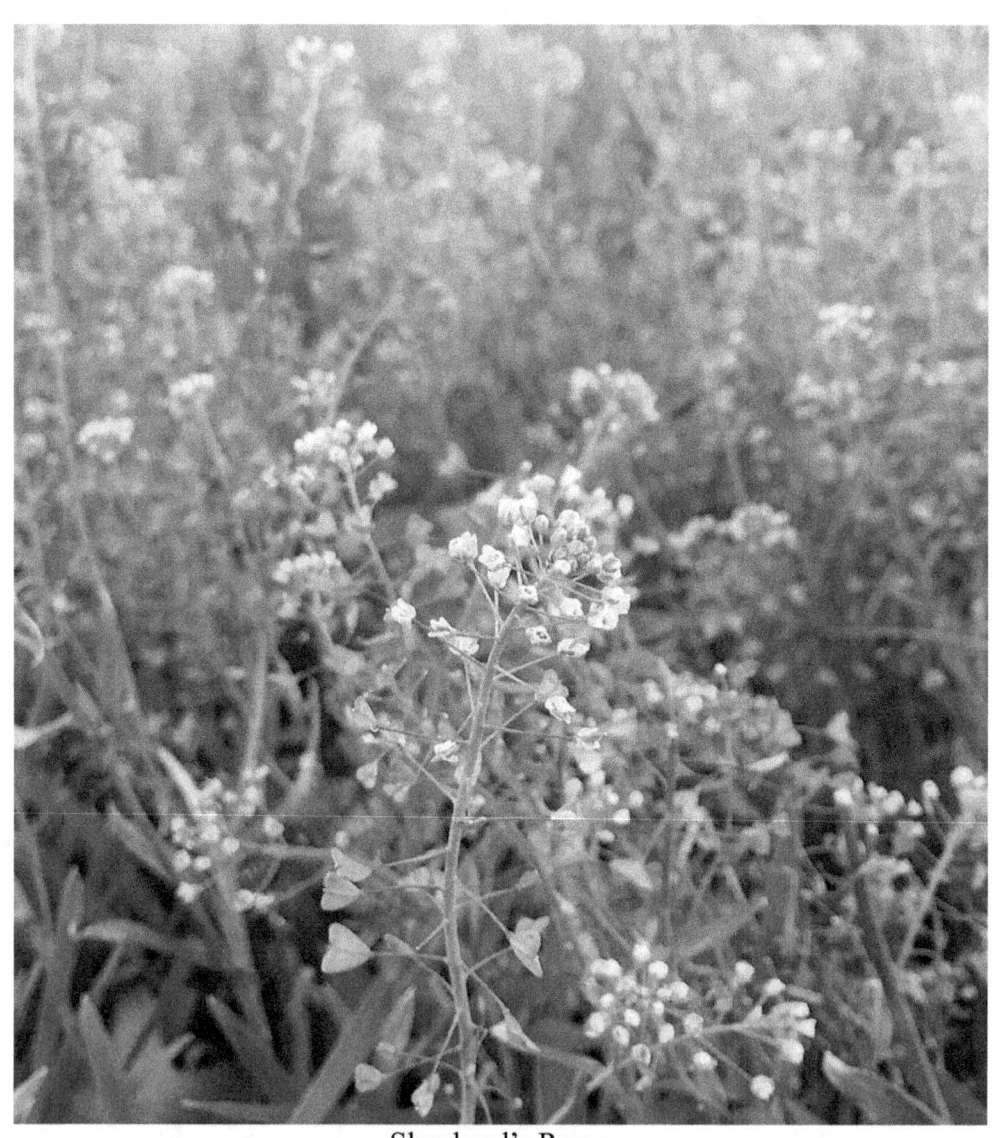
Shepherd's Purse

8.6 Eye injuries and infections

Of all of the senses, I believe the most debilitating in the short term would have to be eyesight. This section will be dealing with any problem affecting the eyes in a first aid type event such as infections, injuries, and conjunctivitis.

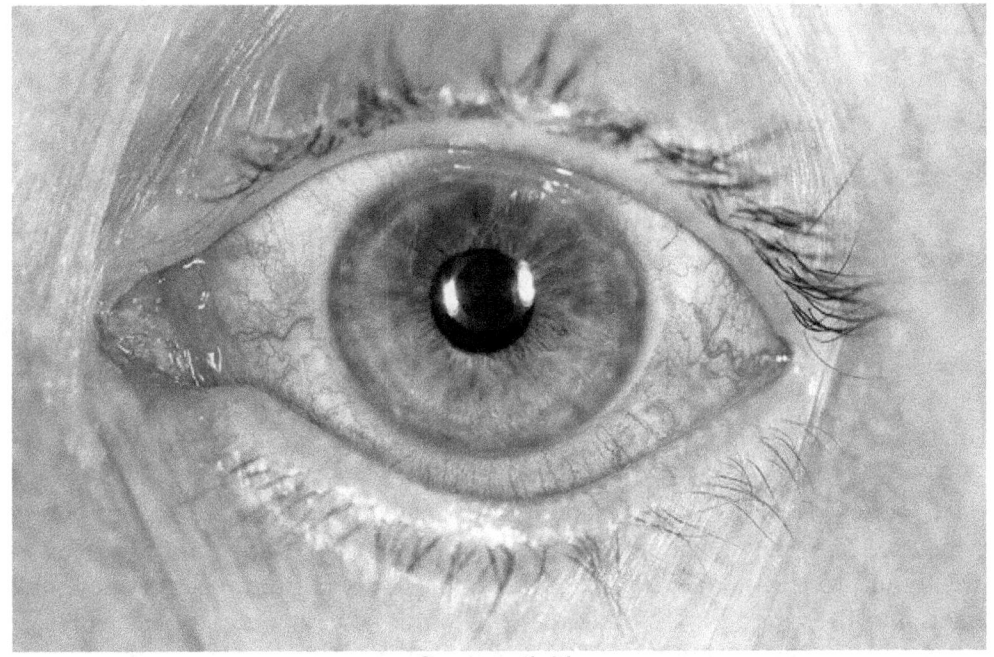

Conjunctivitis

CONJUNCTIVITIS: Also known as pink-eye, this is an infection, usually bacterial, and an inflammation of the conjunctiva. The conjunctiva is the thin clear tissue that lies over the white part of the eye and lines the inside of the eyelid. Children are usually the largest group who are afflicted with this infection.

Several things could be to blame, including:

- Viruses, including the kind that causes the common cold
- Bacteria
- Irritants such as shampoos, dirt, smoke, and pool chlorine
- A reaction to eyedrops
- An allergic reaction to things like pollen, dust, or smoke. Or it could be due to a special type of allergy that affects some people who wear contact lenses.
- Fungi, amoebas, and parasites

For an herbalist, this can be a very easy condition to treat. We prefer this to the use of antibiotics since they will usually destroy the micro-flora in the intestinal tract, thereby suppressing the body's immune system.

HERBAL AIDS FOR CONJUNCTIVITIS AND OTHER INFECTIONS:

Red Raspberry tea: A simple eyewash can be made from this tea and dripped into the eye when cooled. You can also use the cooled teabag after you have made tea with it and place it over the closed eye for about a half an hour, several times a day.

Raw Honey: Raw honey from a compassionate bee keeper is very antibiotic in nature. They have actually taken honey out of pyramids, laid down over two thousands years ago and was still viable. Take a drop of the honey and place into the eye and ask the patient to blink several times. It may take a couple of times a day but the results are amazing.

Mother's milk: Yes, I said mother's milk, human mother's milk. It is very high in natural antibiotics and can clear up a case of pink-eye over night. Use the same as the raw honey described above.

Dr. Christopher's Herbal Eyebright: As stated by Dr. Christopher: "this formula is excellent for helping to brighten and heal the eyes, and it is known to help remove the cataracts and heavy film from the eyes. "I personally have seen patients who needed to wear glasses and were able to give them up after a couple of month of using this eyewash regularly. It is made from bayberry, cayenne, eyebright, golden seal and red raspberry leaves. The formula is as follows or you can purchase it online:

1 part Bayberry bark (Myrica cerifera)
1 part Eyebright (Euphrasia officinalis)
1 part Golden seal root (Hydrastis canadensis)
1 part Red Raspberry leaves (Rubus idaeus)
1/8 part cayenne (Capsicum annuum)

It can be drank as a tea, 1cup twice a day along with using as an eyewash.

To use as an eyewash:
Start each morning by filling up a glass eye cup about two thirds with clean distilled water. Place one drop of the Herbal Eyebright tincture into it. At first it will sting a little so we ask that you start slowly. Now, move the eye cup over the eye socket and tip your head back. Some may spill out so you can do this in the shower or place a towel over you neck for any leakage. Open you eye and look around like you would under water for about 30 to 60 seconds. Now repeat for the other eye but first wash the cup out and start over. This way you lower the risk of passing back and forth bacteria. Do this both in the morning and at night before bed. You can also drink a cup of the tea each time.

As the days or week go by, increase the dosage all the way up to about five drops or more. Again, we have seen wonderful results doing this procedure.

For all of the above protocols: follow until the issue is resolved.

All of the above herbal remedies also work on stys.

Baby Clogged Eye Duct: If your baby has an eye infection which is not gonorrheal you can suspect a plugged tear duct. Many mothers gently massage the area and/or wash it with eyebright and golden seal tea, which sometimes helps open the duct. If it doesn't open after a couple of months, you may wish to go to a good eye doctor for surgical opening of the duct.

Foreign Particles: If you get a foreign particle in your eye, or if your eyes become red and irritated, you can wash them either with Dr. Christopher's Eyewash, being sure to strain the tea carefully through a fine, clean cotton cloth, or a simple tea of red raspberry leaves. These teas help astringe and heal the irritated surface.

Some testimonials from Dr. Christopher and my practice:

1.) **Subretinal Hemorrhage**: My right eye went bad last January, diagnosed as "subretinal hemorrhage" which left me with probably 20-30% vision. Since using Eyebright Comb. [Herbal Eyebright], I now have 70 or 80% vision. Miracle Medicines-God's wonderful herbs.

2.) **Eye Pain**: The eyebright combination [Herbal Eyebright] has brought good results for a very severe pain behind one eye. (I have had this for over two years and the doctors have been unable to find the cause).

3.) In my practice I had a gentleman come in to the clinic complaining of having a restriction on his drivers license requiring him to wear eyeglasses. He used the Herbal eyewash formula for 60 days. When he returned to the DMV he was retested and passed the eye exam. The restriction was removed from his license.

4.) A mother brought her ten year old girl into the clinic one day with a very serious case of pink-eye. The school had sent her home. After using the eyewash for just a couple of days, the eye had healed enough where she was able to go back to school.

CHAPTER 9

ADVANCED FIRST-AID

9.1 Major Bleeding/Shock/Deep Cuts and Wounds

In the previous chapter we discussed coping with bleeding injuries, mainly minor and external. In this section we will cover how to treat more serious injuries such as internal, bleeding during labor and more serious external wounds when the opportunity for emergency medical care is not available.

When coping with a significant injury resulting in high blood loss shock is a very significant possibility and this along can kill a patient. It is important that we know the signs of shock and how to treat them.

SHOCK : SIGNS & SYMPTOMS

- ✚ **Discolourisation of Face**
- ✚ **Loss of Power**
- ✚ **Slow/weak Pulse**
- ✚ **Cold Sweating**
- ✚ **Irregular Breathing/Shallow breathing**
- ✚ **Nausea & Giddiness**
- ✚ **Clammy & Sandy Skin**
- ✚ **Fall in Temperature**

According to the Mayo Clinic: Shock is a critical condition brought on by the sudden drop in blood flow through the body. Shock may result from trauma, heatstroke, blood loss, an allergic reaction, severe infection, poisoning, severe burns or other causes. When a person is in shock, his or her organs aren't getting enough blood or oxygen. If untreated, this can lead to permanent organ damage or even death.

Signs and symptoms of shock vary depending on circumstances and may include:

- Cool, clammy skin
- Pale or ashen skin
- Bluish tinge to lips or fingernails (or gray in the case of dark complexions)
- Rapid pulse
- Rapid breathing
- Nausea or vomiting
- Enlarged pupils
- Weakness or fatigue
- Dizziness or fainting
- Changes in mental status or behavior, such as anxiousness or agitation.

Treatment for shock needs to be immediate. Take the following steps:

- Lay the person down and elevate the legs and feet slightly, unless you think this may cause pain or further injury.
- Keep the person still and don't move him or her unless necessary.
- Begin CPR if the person shows no signs of life, such as not breathing, coughing or moving.
- Loosen tight clothing and, if needed, cover the person with a blanket to prevent chilling.
- Don't let the person eat or drink anything.
- If the person vomits or begins bleeding from the mouth, and no spinal injury is suspected, turn him or her onto a side to prevent choking.

HERBAL AIDS FOR SHOCK AND MAJOR BLEEDING:

Here again, we return to that miracle herb ... cayenne. It is useful for both shock and bleeding injuries. As quoted from Dr. Christopher: "General Instructions For Shock: When a person goes into shock, the administration of medicinal aids orally will often be difficult or impossible. In this case an anus injection (or enema) which will cause relaxation is applicable. Use one cup (to a pint maximum) of catnip, peppermint, skullcap, spearmint, or Valerian.

Massage the abdomen and parts of the spine with Lobelia externally and make sure that the patient gets undisturbed rest. Cayenne should be taken internally to help equalize the blood pressure and insure that the internal functions will remain stabilized during the intense systemal distress."

When shock is caused by hemorrhaging: "Hemorrhage throws many people into shock and can bring on death very rapidly. If the wound is small, the blood usually coagulates and the area seals itself, but if the rupture is large, some herbal aid is needed. The first thing one should think about is cayenne as quickly as possible. Using one teaspoon to the cup, as hot as can be taken without scalding. This will help stop any hemorrhage, internal or external, by the time a person can count to ten. If the rupture is external and cayenne is not available, Comfrey placed over the wound will stop bleeding quickly."

The **Bach Flower Rescue Remedy** also works very well for shock to aid the patient to quickly recover. Give a few drops at the time of the incident.

Cayenne for serious wounds: In wounds, though the wound is cut and exposed to the bone, that wound may be filled with cayenne pepper (and if cayenne is not available, black pepper) and it will heal beautifully and stop the bleeding. Many people, when they seen the skin ruddier by cayenne, believe that the skin is irritated; but cayenne is a counter-irritant; there is no itching involved with it. What cayenne is actually doing is bringing the blood to the surface to take away any toxic poisons, or to start the healing; so the redness comes to the skin from the blood that has rushed to the surface to assist in carrying off wastes

Aloe Vera: Other external uses for the herb include treatment for all kinds of wounds--scrapes, cuts, etc. The gel seems to mildly kill the germs on the surface and promote healing. The herb is high in calcium, which reduces bleeding with its coagulating action, at the same time helping to stimulate circulation of blood in the surrounding areas to bring oxygen to the surface.

Ulcers: We need to go to the cause of ulcers and eliminate those but we can begin by relieving the pain and healing the tissues. Cayenne pepper should be taken by the teaspoon (start with 1/4 tsp. three times a day and work up to 1 teaspoonful three times a day). The cayenne pepper will even cauterize a bleeding ulcer.

FOR TREATING WOUNDS AND ENCOURAGING HEALING:

Having covered chock and bleeding, what do we do about the actual healing of the wound? Again, these are suggestions for folks without access to a qualified healthcare provider.

I mentioned earlier about using holistic medications such as **Herbadyne** and the **Green Salve.** They both easily apply here but I would like to give a word of warning. I do not apply a healing salve too quickly to a deep, open wound. The salves we are discussing here are very fast acting and can cause a wound to seal very quickly. If the wound was not properly cleansed first and not had an antiseptic applied first than dirt and bacteria could get trapped in the closing wound.

The first thing of course is to stem the bleeding as shown above. Next, clean the wound thoroughly with water or Hydrogen Peroxide. It is at this point you can then liberally use something like our Herbadyne formula. It will most likely sting but it is doing it's job. I would not use a strong healing salve for at least a day, to give the wound a chance to clean out.

One of the best formulas I have worked with for quick wound healing is Dr. Christopher's B, F and C. You can make it into a salve, capsules, syrup, shampoo, oil, etc. It stands for Bone, Flesh and Cartilage and it is meant to heal each of those tissues very quickly. You can purchase it online or you can make it with the included formula here.

6 Parts Oak Bark (Quercus alba)
3 Parts Marshmallow Root (Althaea officinalis)
3 Parts Mullein Herb (Verbascum thapsus)
2 Parts Wormwood (Artemisia absinthium)
1 Part Lobelia (Lobelia inflata)
1 Part Skullcap (Scutellaria lateriflora)
6 Parts Comfrey Root (Symphytum officinalis)
3 Parts Walnut Bark or leaves (Juglans nigra)
3 Parts Gravel root (Eupatorium purpureum)

This combination has saved many, many lives and limbs. If you will look back at page 17 you will see the foot that was healed, in part, with this combination because of the Comfrey in it. I have seen cases where deep, serious wounds healed with no scarring afterwards.

For very serious wounds, I would take the B, F and C in both an oral and an external treatment. During the beginning of the healing process the usual dosage is 5 capsules five times a day until the worse is over. It can take days or weeks, depending on the severity of the wound. At the same time I would also apply the B, F and C as a salve to the wound, after a day or two of using something like the Herbadyne as an antiseptic. After a couple of days you can start using the B, F and C salve. Make sure to apply the Herbadyne or some other natural antiseptic first and then the salve on top of it. Bandage over the salve. Change the dressing and reapply the antiseptic and the salve each day.

DOGS LEGS SAVED:

I have also seen the above salve used on other animals such as dogs. In two separate cases, I have seen dogs destined by their vets to have a leg amputated due to gaping open wounds. On both occasions, the caregivers chose to use the B, F and C salves on them and the legs completely healed. Both vets were quite amazed at the results.

Testimonials from Dr. Christopher:

1.) Cayenne and the Gunshot Wound: Once a child was shot in the abdomen; a bullet hit the spine, ricocheted, and made a second wound leaving the body. One of Dr. Christopher's herbal students, living next door, heard the shot and raced over, as she knew that the parents were not home and that the children, ages eight and four, would not be shooting guns. There was the eight-year-old gushing blood out both sides. She ran to the cabinet and mixed a tablespoonful of cayenne in a glass of water; she poured it down the boy and immediately called the ambulance, which was eighteen miles away. The emergency room attendant said that the boy would probably bleed to death, being that the distance was so great.

The ambulance arrived and rushed the child (who had been playing "Cops and Robbers" with his father's pistol, which he had found under the pillow of the bed, to the Primary Children's Hospital eighteen miles away. When he arrived, he was the center of attraction, not because his case was so dangerous, but because he was chatting a mile a minute--and there was no bleeding. The bleeding had stopped by the time they arrived at the hospital. The chief doctor said to the parents, "I have seen many accident victims in my life, but this is the first time in such an emergency operation that I have opened an abdomen to find no blood, except for a small amount that was there before the bleeding stopped so quickly. This has saved your boy's life."

2.) Stomach Ulcer: I had symptoms of a stomach ulcer and I drank the Cayenne Pepper and now I have no more symptoms. Thank you again for your information on Cayenne and how it works for bleeding and heart attacks.

3.) Cayenne: A person in our audience told how he had cut deeply with a sharp instrument the inside of his hand, fingers and palm. The blood spurted out in streams. He poured a large amount of cayenne pepper into the wound, and within seconds the blood flow slowed down to congealed dripping and the bleeding stopped entirely before many seconds had passed. With a goodly amount of cayenne covering the wound, he then wrapped it. He was so excited about the rapid results he could hardly wait for the regular herb meeting. But, as he said, the "punch line" was lost, because instead of a nasty ragged scar to show how severely he had been hurt, the area was healed and there was no scar.

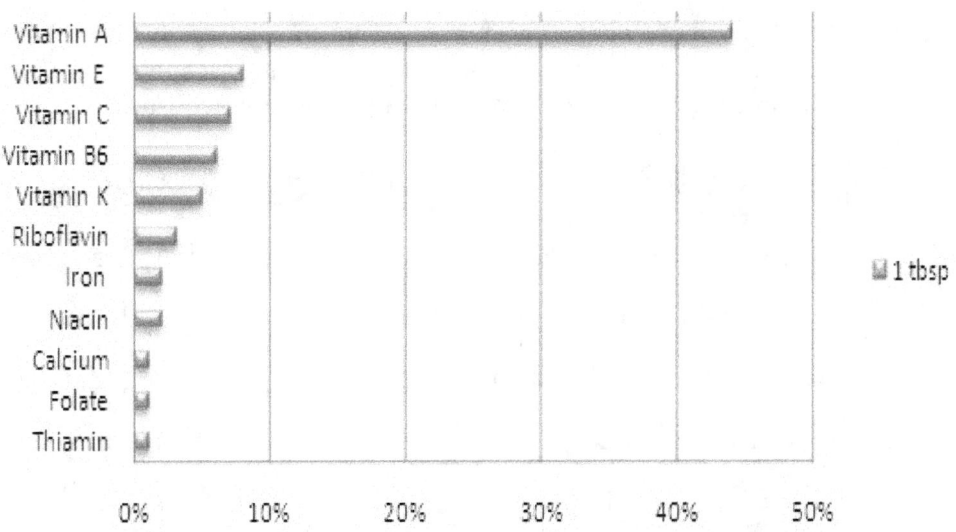

9.2 Poisoning

Unfortunately, this is an all too common occurrence in many households across America. In 2017, the 55 U.S. poison control centers provided telephone guidance for nearly 2.12 million human poison exposures.

	Year: 2017
Human Poison Exposures	2,115,186
Animal Poison Exposures	51,164
Confirmed Non-Exposures	5,523
Info Calls - Drug ID	96,221
Info Calls - Other	339,319
Total	2,607,413

According to poison.org: While young children (younger than 6 years) comprise a disproportionate percentage of the cases, poisoning affects ALL age groups, from infants to seniors. Peak poisoning frequency occurs in one and two year olds, but poisonings in teens and adults are more serious. Notice that the greater proportion of males in poison exposures occurring in children younger than 13 years switches to a female predominance in teens and adults.

Across all ages, there were 640 poison exposures reported per 100,000 population. The highest incidence occurred in one and two year olds (7,542 and 7,270 exposures/100,000 children in the respective age groups). For ages 50 years or older, 250 exposures were reported per 100,000 population.

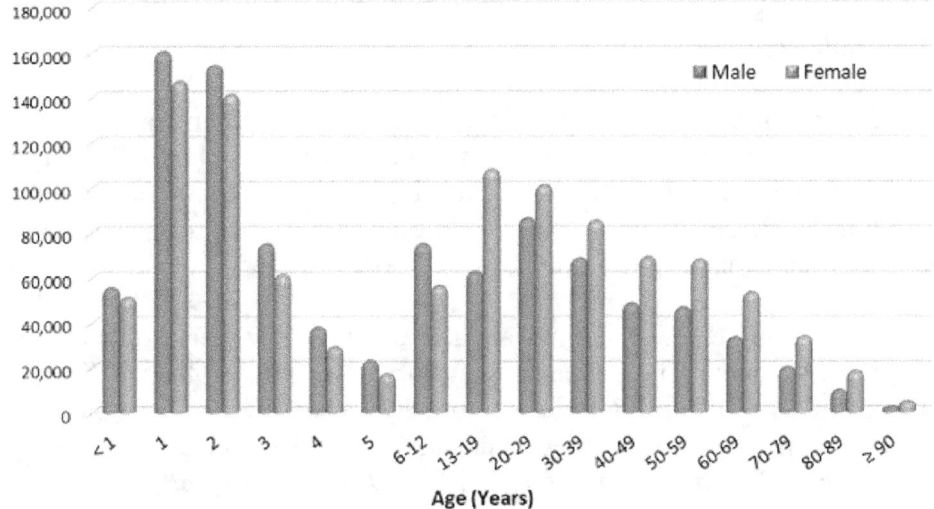

The most common substances involved in childhood poisonings reported:

- Cosmetics and Personal care products
- Cleaning substances
- Analgesics
- Foreign bodies/toys/Misc.
- Topical preparations
- Antihistamines
- Vitamins
- Pesticides
- Dietary supplements
- Plants

The most common substances involved in adult poisonings reported:

- Analgesics
- Sedative/Hypnotics/Anti-psychotics
- Antidepressants
- Cardiovascular drugs
- Household cleaning substances
- Alcohols
- Anticonvulsants

- Pesticides
- Stimulants and street drugs
- Antihistamines

What is also interesting is that the leading cause of children's poisoning in the 1990s was Flintstones vitamins with iron. They taste and look like candy so children were eating as such and the high iron content was poisoning them. I have in my practice treated children for iron toxicity from well meaning parents thinking if a little is good, more is better.

A significant number of poisonings are also due to heavy metal toxicity from such metals as lead. The scope of that subject is greater than a first aid treatment. If you would like to learn more about how to cure chronic heavy metal poisoning than please check out our book ***A Complete Body Repair, Healing Candida, Parasite and Heavy Metal Toxicity Naturally***.

The type of first aid for poisoning varies depending on the type of chemical ingested. Overall, to start with, a very good rule of thumb is to not induce vomiting unless you have been instructed otherwise by a qualified healthcare provider. It used to a be standard decades ago to induce vomiting but it has been found that it can greatly increase the damage depending on the type of poison. So for now, no inducing your patient to vomit. We will work instead in strengthening the body's own defenses and neutralizing the poison.

Let's start with the basics. According to PSEP (Pesticide Safety Education Program):

Poison on the Skin
The sooner the poison is washed off the patient, the less the injury.

- Remove clothing and drench skin with water (shower, hose, faucet, pond, ditch).
- Cleanse skin and hair thoroughly with soap and water. (Don't abrade or injure the skin while washing.)
- Dry and wrap in a blanket

Warning: Do not allow any of the pesticide to get on you while you are helping the victim.

Chemical Burns of the Skin

- Remove contaminated clothing.
- Wash the skin with large quantities of cold running water.
- Immediately cover loosely with a clean, soft cloth.
- Avoid use of ointments, greases, powders, and other drugs in the first aid treatment of chemical burns.

Poison in the Eye

It is very important to wash the eye as quickly, but as gently, as possible.

- Hold eyelids open, wash eyes with a gentle stream of clean running water at body temperature.
- Continue washing for 15 minutes or more.
- Do not use chemicals or drugs in wash water. They may increase the extent of injury.

Inhaled Poisons (Dust, Vapors, Gases)

If victim is in an enclosed area use an air-supplied respirator to get to him.

- Carry patient (do not let him walk) to fresh air immediately.
- Open all doors and windows.
- Loosen all tight clothing.
- Apply artificial respiration if breathing has stopped or is irregular.
- Keep patient as quiet as possible.
- If patient is convulsing, watch his breathing and protect him from falling and striking his head. Pull his chin forward so his tongue does not block his air passage.
- Do not give alcohol in any form.

Swallowed Poisons

The most important decision you have to make when aiding a person who has swallowed a pesticide or poison is whether to induce vomiting or not.

The decision must be made quickly and accurately; the victim's life may depend on it. Usually it is best to get rid of the swallowed poison fast. But: **NEVER** induce vomiting if the victim is unconscious or is in convulsions. The victim could choke to death on vomitus.

Find out what poison has been ingested. **NEVER** induce vomiting if the victim has swallowed a corrosive poison. A corrosive poison is a strong acid or alkali (base) such as dinoseb (DN Compounds). The victim will complain of severe pain and have signs of severe mouth and throat burns. A corrosive poison wil burn the throat and mouth as severely coming up as it did going down.

Most labels on emulsifiable concentrate and solution formulations suggest the victim should not have vomiting induced. However, when the toxicity of the pesticide is marked, its removal may be essential.

Corrosive Poisons

The best first aid is to dilute the poison as quickly as possible. For acids or alkalis (bases), give the patient water or preferably a plant based milk - one (1) cup for victims under five (5) years; or one (1) to two (2) glasses for patients over five (5) years. The plant milk is better than water because it dilutes and helps neutralize the poison. Water only dilutes the poison.

It is very important that the victim get to a hospital without delay. **DO NOT INDUCE OR ENCOURAGE VOMITING FOR CORROSIVE POISONS!**

Activated Charcoal

After first-aid suggestions for noncorrosive poisons have been followed and medical help is delayed due to travel or other reasons, activated charcoal may be administered to hopefully absorb the remaining poison. It does not absorb all poisons and a rather large amount may be required for it to be effective. For example: it takes 1-1/2 ounces of charcoal powder (about 10 grams) to bind 3 adult aspirin. Mix the charcoal with water into a thick soup for the victim to drink.

HERBAL AIDES:

Milk Thistle: Milk Thistle is known around the world as one of the best natural aids for protecting and healing the liver. It is best known for it's ability to cure the Death cap mushroom poison. According to David Hoffmann, he suggests that the best results with using Milk thistle are found in toxic metabolic hepatitis and cirrhosis, in that it shortens the length of viral hepatitis, minimizes complications and also protects the liver against problems arising from surgery. He writes, "This all goes to make it an excellent remedy to use in the prevention and treatments of many liver disorders. The earlier treatment is commenced the better the prognosis but effective treatment is possible at virtually every stage."

DOSAGE: Milk thistle can be taken in the powdered form, also as an infusion, a decoction, glycerine extract, and also alcohol extract, with the alcohol extract being the strongest.

In the powdered form a dosage of two to four grams three times per day is normal. For the infusion use one teaspoonful of the powdered herb to 150 ml of boiling distilled water left to infuse for ten minutes and drink this three times per day. For the decoction use three teaspoonfuls of the seeds to half a pint of distilled water and simmer for about twenty minutes, drink this three times per day. In the case of the glycerine and alcohol extract take 2.5 mls three times per day. In the case of poisoning where there is need to act quickly take 1:1 liquid extract at doses of 10 mls three or more times per day.

In severe poisoning cases, I would use a dropperfull every hour for 8 to 10 hours.

Dr. Christopher's Liver and Gallbladder Formula: This is a tried and true formula we have used in the clinic for over 20 years. It helps tone and cleanse the liver. It is best used in conjunction with other holistic aids during poisoning, though we have seen it effective when we had nothing else to use. On one occasion, our cat had eaten a poisonous animal such as a toad. He was almost dead when we found him, lethargic and barely breathing. He would take no water and could not lift his head and was quite limp. We used an eyedropper and gave him water and the Liver and Gallbladder Formula.

In this case we gave him an eyedropper full every half an hour. All together it took about two hours but eventually he started to move around and was able to get up and quickly gained a full recovery.

The formula is

3 parts Barberry (Berberis vulgaris)

1 part Wild yam (Dioscorea villosa)

1 part Cramp bark (Viburnum trilobum)

1 part Fennel seed (Foeniculum vulgare)

1 part Ginger (Zingiber officinalis)

1 part Catnip (Nepeta cataria)

1 part Peppermint (Mentha piperita)

Plantain (Plantago major): It has been used historically as an excellent aid against such poisons as snake bit and black widow. Plantain is also used as an antivenomous herb in its role as a blood cleanser. Terry Willard, author of *Edible and Medicinal Plants of the Rocky Mountains and Neighbouring Territories*, states that it is good to draw out the poison of snake bites. It is an excellent choice for poisonous bites and stings of scorpions and insects.

Plantain is #1 in the field of blood poisoning treatment. You can see the healing at work. Swelling goes down and the "red" line recedes. Limbs poisoned can be saved using this herb. It is used as a poultice on the outside and taken as a tea on the inside.

It is best in this case to take as a tincture or a tea orally to get it into the system quickly. The tea is made with one teaspoon to a cup of water or a tablespoon to a pint. Drink at least five cups a day during an episode of poising. It the poison is from a bite or a sting, then also put a poultice of plantain on the wound to aid in drawing out the poison.

An incident that occurred with me several years was helped greatly from this plant. I had been bitten on the hand by a spider and it became a nasty looking ulcer and infected. I made a poultice of the fresh leaves (can be found in most yards that haven't had all of the "weeds" removed) and left it on over night. Very quickly I noticed the pain diminishing. By morning, I removed the poultice and the infection had been completely drawn out the wound was sealing. A truly amazing wonder of a plant, and considered such a "weed" by so many.

Dr. Christopher's Blood Stream Formula: According to Dr. Christopher, the Blood Purifying Formula containing red clover, chaparral, licorice root, poke root, peach bark, Oregon grape root, stillingia, prickly ash bark, burdock root, and buckthorn bark. This formula creates, not only a generalized blood purifier, but also includes a group of herbs that aid in building strength and cleaning out the entire body, by helping break loose toxic deposits and flush them out, and also acting as a food for the organs.

DOSAGE: During a poisoning event this formula, used in conjunction with any of the above methods will aid in speeding up the healing process by getting the poisons out of the blood more quickly. During a crisis, I would use one dropperful every hour for six to eight hours, until the crisis has passed.

The formula:

2 parts Red Clover blossoms (Trifolium pratense)

1 part Chaparral (Larrea tridentata)

1 part Licorice root (Glycyrrhiza glabra)

1 part Poke root (Phytolacca americana)

1 part Peach bark (Prunus persica)

1 part Oregon grape root (Mahonia aquifolium)

1 part Stillingia (Stillingia sylvatica)

1 part Cascara sagrada (Rhamnus purshiana)

1 part Sarsaparilla (Smilax aspera)

1 part Prickly ash bark (Zanthoxylum americanum)

1 part Burdock root (Arctium lappa)

1 part Buckthorn bark (Rhamnus frangula)

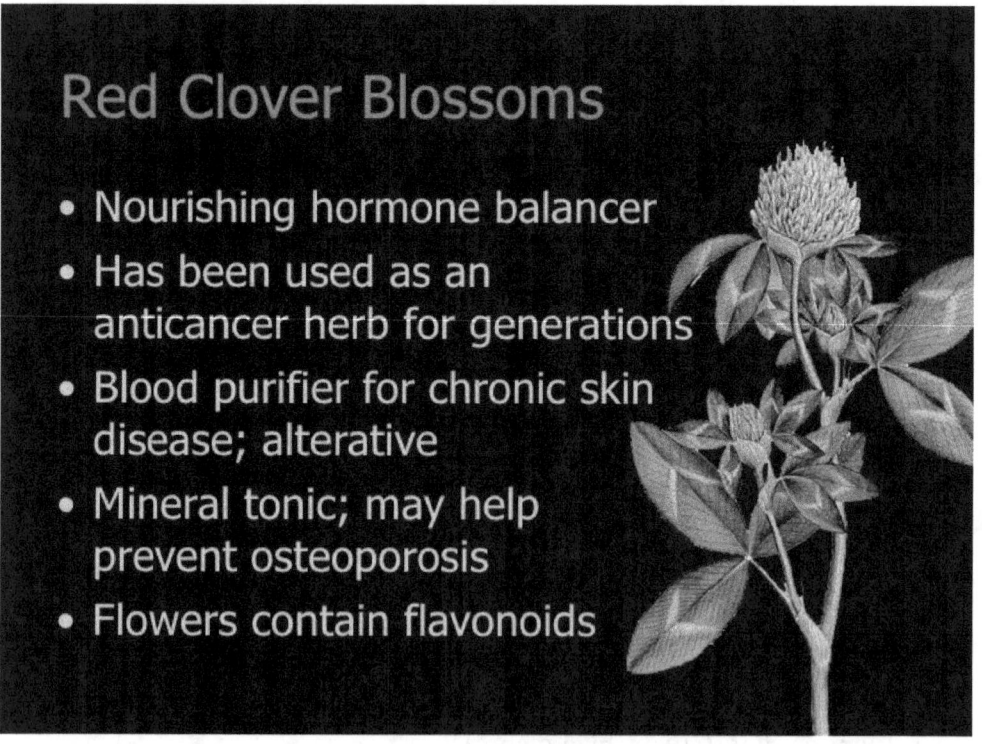

Red Clover Blossoms

- Nourishing hormone balancer
- Has been used as an anticancer herb for generations
- Blood purifier for chronic skin disease; alterative
- Mineral tonic; may help prevent osteoporosis
- Flowers contain flavonoids

9.3 Broken bones

Broken bones rank towards the top of some of the most painful and serious emergencies you may encounter and one of the scariest without a qualified healthcare provider present. It can be from simple fall off a chair to hiking though the mountains with no one around. This is again one of the those situations where it is often best to get to a hospital but we will cover what you can do without such access. We will also discuss what you can do if you have received emergency room treatment and would like to heal faster.

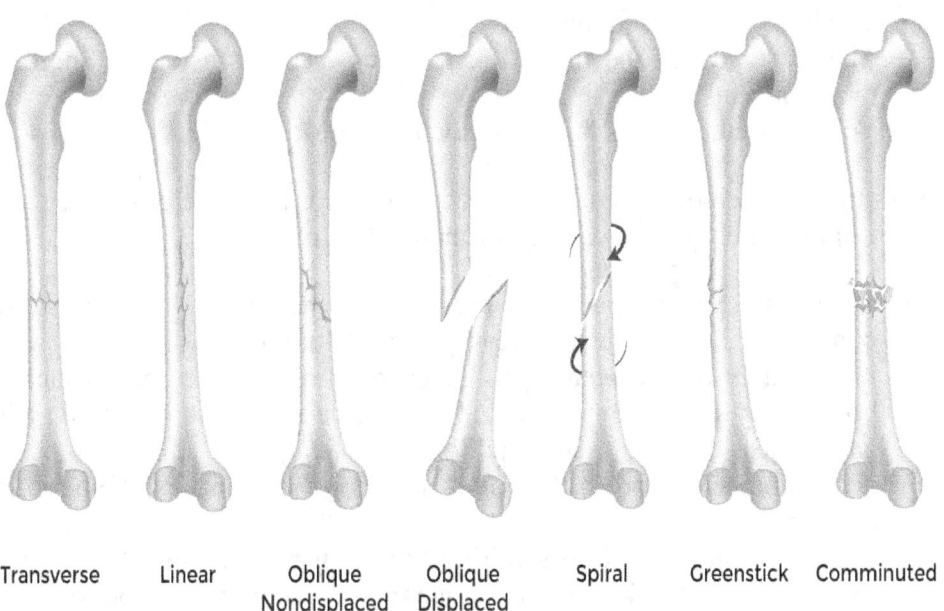

Transverse | Linear | Oblique Nondisplaced | Oblique Displaced | Spiral | Greenstick | Comminuted

Types of broken bones

BASIC BROKEN BONE FIRST AID:

According to the Mayo clinic:

A fracture is a broken bone. It requires medical attention. If the broken bone is the result of major trauma or injury, call 911 or your local emergency number.
Also call for emergency help if:

- The person is unresponsive, isn't breathing or isn't moving. Begin CPR if there's no breathing or heartbeat.
- There is heavy bleeding.
- Even gentle pressure or movement causes pain.
- The limb or joint appears deformed.
- The bone has pierced the skin.
- The extremity of the injured arm or leg, such as a toe or finger, is numb or bluish at the tip.
- You suspect a bone is broken in the neck, head or back.

Don't move the person except if necessary to avoid further injury. Take these actions immediately while waiting for medical help:

- **Stop any bleeding.** Apply pressure to the wound with a sterile bandage, a clean cloth or a clean piece of clothing.
- **Immobilize the injured area.** Don't try to realign the bone or push a bone that's sticking out back in. If you've been trained in how to splint and professional help isn't readily available, apply a splint to the area above and below the fracture sites. Padding the splints can help reduce discomfort.
- **Apply ice packs to limit swelling and help relieve pain.** Don't apply ice directly to the skin. Wrap the ice in a towel, piece of cloth or some other material.
- **Treat for shock.** If the person feels faint or is breathing in short, rapid breaths, lay the person down with the head slightly lower than the trunk and, if possible, elevate the legs. We discussed this in the section on Bleeding.

HERBAL AIDS:

Dr. Christopher's B, F and C Formula: This is by far the best formula I have used for encouraging rapid healing of a broken bone. As stated earlier; B, F and C stands for Bone, Flesh and Cartilage. The formula is described in the section **Major Bleeding/Shock/Deep Cuts and Wounds.**

Dr. Christopher often recommended a calcium tea with Comfrey to help with mending broken bones. An example was:

Comfrey Tea and Organic Calcium: After the doctor has set the bone, drink three or more cups of Comfrey tea each day--the more the better. With each cup of tea take the calcium combination. This is the formula:

6 parts Horsetail grass
4 parts Comfrey root
3 parts Oat straw
1 part Lobelia

For children old enough to take capsules, use two capsules or more, three times in a day. As suggested, take these capsules with the Comfrey tea. Mix the powder with blackstrap molasses, if it is hard to swallow the capsules.

Broken Bones After Being Set: After a doctor has set the bone, drink three or more cups of Complete Tissue & Bone and/or Comfrey tea or green drink per day. With each cup take two or more capsules of the Calc formula.

Here was a testimonial given to Dr. Christopher quite a few years ago: *"Over the years of practice I have had a number of patients who have had broken bones from osteoporosis. One case was a woman in her middle eighties with a fractured hip. After three months in a cast it showed no sign of healing, any more than two pieces of stick growing together. This woman was frightened because she was told that if the hip bones did not knit after putting on another cast for three months, they would cut her leg open and use stainless steel rods, bolts and nuts to make it possible for her to at least get around on crutches. This was in the early sixties and not much Comfrey was available then. The lady's daughter was in one of my classes, and we asked the students to help out by donating as much Comfrey as they could. We had enough donated from the class members that the patient had from a pint to a quart of Comfrey green drink or Comfrey tea each day, six days a week, week after week. At the end of this "three months," the cast was removed and the doctors were amazed, because during the first three months were was "no knitting" of the bone even evident, but with the Comfrey being taken orally during the next three-month period the leg was healed. The daughter told us her mother was out square dancing within a couple of weeks after the cast was removed!*

Since this case was so outstanding we have had a formula developed called "bone, flesh and cartilage."[Complete Tissue & Bone] This formula has done miraculous things with broken backs, legs, hips, etc. This formula has been used to help with curvature of the spine, polio, multiple sclerosis, and muscular dystrophy, stroke and arthritis of the bone. This formula is used externally as well as orally and has brought tremendously fast results."

If taken as capsules for mending a broken bone I have found that 3 capsules 4 times day works well and for a more rapid healing I would use 5 capsules 5 times a day. I have seen broken bones healed in a third to half of the time usually seen in conventional medicine.

Comfrey: If you do not have access to the above formulas then Comfrey alone can do the job. It has a history of thousands of years in promoting bone health when a fracture has occurred. It can be made as a poultice, a fomentation, taken as a tea or in capsule form.

The roots are more potent than the leaves but if you cannot get them than the leaves will help:

Decoction 2 fluid ounces three times daily.
Fluid extract ½-2 teaspoonfuls.
Infusion 1 cupful, 3 times daily.
Powder 2 #00 capsules or 1 teaspoonful
Tincture ½-1 teaspoonful (fluid teaspoon)

9.4 Heart Attack/Strokes

HEART ATTACK FACTS:

According to the CDC; **every 40 seconds**, someone in the United States has a heart attack.

A heart attack, also called a myocardial infarction, occurs when a part of the heart muscle doesn't receive enough blood flow. The more time that passes without treatment to restore blood flow, the greater the damage to the heart muscle.

Every year, about **790,000 Americans** have a heart attack. Of these cases

- 580,000 are a first heart attack.
- 210,000 happen to people who have already had a first heart attack.[1]

One of 5 heart attacks is silent—the damage is done, but the person is not aware of it.

The five major symptoms of a heart attack are

- Pain or discomfort in the jaw, neck, or back.
- Feeling weak, light-headed, or faint.
- Chest pain or discomfort.
- Pain or discomfort in arms or shoulder.
- Shortness of breath.

Other symptoms of a heart attack could include unusual or unexplained tiredness and nausea or vomiting. Women are more likely to have these other symptoms.

STROKE FACTS:

Stroke is the fifth leading cause of death in the United States and is a major cause of serious disability for adults. About **795,000** people in the United States have a stroke each year.

Stroke Statistics

- Stroke kills about **140,000** Americans each year—that's **1 out of every 20 deaths**.
- Someone in the United States has a stroke every **40 seconds**. Every **4 minutes**, someone dies of stroke.
- Every year, more than **795,000 people** in the United States have a stroke. About 610,000 of these are first or new strokes.
- About 185,000 strokes—**nearly 1 of 4**—are in people who have had a previous stroke.
- About **87%** of all strokes are ischemic strokes, in which blood flow to the brain is blocked.
- Stroke costs the United States an estimated **$34 billion** each year. This total includes the cost of health care services, medicines to treat stroke, and missed days of work.
- Stroke is a leading cause of serious long-term disability. Stroke reduces mobility in more than half of stroke survivors age 65 and over.

Unfortunately, the average person is completely unaware that they are even at risk so they are caught by surprise when it happens. In most cases, this means they are completely unprepared. What can we do for ourselves and our family members to help them have more than the "four golden minutes" needed to save their lives in the event of a heart attack or stroke?

As stated before, we return to our favorite herb for emergencies ... Cayenne! Not too surprised are you after reading this whole book? There is NO better herb that can be used for this issues than capsicum annum (cayenne).

We discussed this in some detail earlier but I will detail a few more facts and what you can do in an emergency.

A common protocol recommended by Dr. Christopher and one I have used in my practice is as follows:

Heart Attack: Prop up the patient and pour hot cayenne tea down, (use a teaspoonful of cayenne in a cup of hot water), and have the patient drink the full cup. and the attack will stop immediately. We have been called in the middle of the night so many times. A teaspoon of cayenne should bring the patient out of the heart attack. In case cayenne is not around and you have a heart attack, the dosage on black pepper can be tripled and used.

I have personally seen this technique work and save lives. It will also work on a stroke victim if you get them to take it. If not, I have seen where you can get cayenne tincture or the water with cayenne in it, in an eyedropper (plastic so they don't bite down on it and hurt themselves) and place it on their tongue. The reaction is pretty quick and it can save lives.

As mentioned before, this is due to the fact that cayenne can cause an equalization of blood pressure throughout the body momentarily which in turn takes the pressure off the heart or brain.

Please consider always having a bottle of cayenne tincture available for emergencies. As a tincture it can last for many, many years stored in a cool, dark place such as a medicine cabinet, a purse, etc.

Hawthorne berry Syrup: This is a great herb which has been used historically for heart and circulatory repair. It has been used for thousands of years for such issues as Congestive Heart Failure, arrhythmia, etc. But it also can work on a heart attack. A testimonial given to Dr. Christopher stated:

"One doctor who had learned the formula for Hawthorn berry syrup from Dr. Christopher raised his hand after a lecture to tell the following story. He had gone on a house call in response to a call about a heart attack, one so serious that the family was afraid that death was imminent. The doctor had no cayenne in his bag and the family had no cayenne; the doctor began to panic. He remembered that he had a bottle of Hawthorn berry syrup with him. The usual dose is a half-teaspoonful, but the doctor thought a little more might help, so he gave the patient a full tablespoonful. The patient drank it down, sat right up, and said, "Well, I feel okay". The doctor checked him with the stethoscope and the heart sounded alright. As the doctor said, "Talk about quick relief!"

STOP HEART ATTACK WITH CAYENNE PEPPER

CAYENNE PEPPER   HOT WATER

Dr. John Christopher: "In 35 years of practice I have never on house calls lost one heart attack patient. The reason is if they are still breathing --I pour 1 tsp of cayenne in a cup of hot water, and within minutes they are up and around."

NOTE:
First the Cayenne pepper must be at least 90,000 heat units or 90,000(H.U) to be able to stop a heart.

- If the cayenne is at least 90,000 H.U. and the person is still conscious, the recommendation is to mix 1 tsp of cayenne powder in a glass of warm water, and give it to the person to drink.

- If the person is unconscious then the recommendation is to use a cayenne extract (at least 90,000 H.U), and put 2 full droppers underneath their tongue.

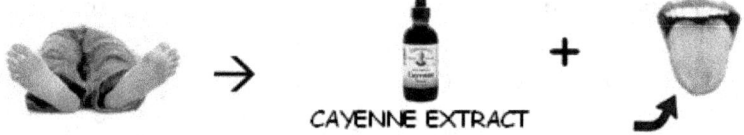

CAYENNE EXTRACT

9.5 Pain Management

One of the most important aspects of treating a patient in an emergency situation is pain management. Without this it can often be difficult to care for an injured patient when they are not able to relax and give in to the care. It can also lead a patient further into shock.

Within the holistic, natural world, most of the best pain killers are illegal so we have to make do with what is available to us. The good news is that there are some very good options for relieving pain.

HERBAL AIDS:

Bugleweed (Lycopus virginicus):

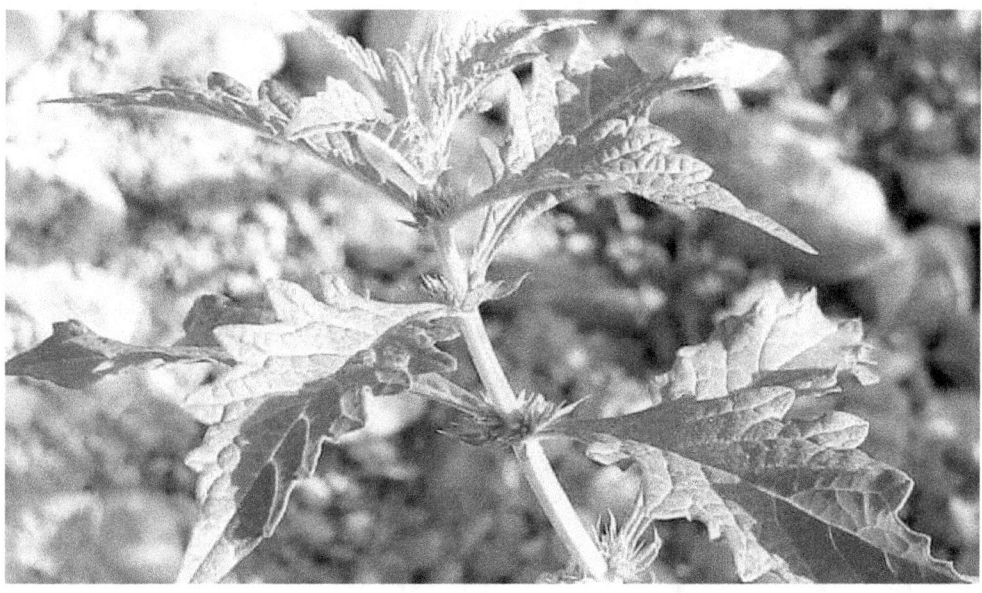

Known botanically as *Lycopus virginicus,* this is a perennial plant that generally thrives in damp regions. The herb actually belongs to the mint family but lacks the familiar minty odor of real mint. Some of its most common uses include treating respiratory illness and bringing balance to the hormones. It's use in this case is it's ability to be slight narcotic. It can be used as a great pain reliever.

I have a personal story with Bugleweed. Many years ago I was scheduled to have all of my wisdom teeth removed along with a cyst that had been caused by the pressure of one of the teeth. Knowing that I would not use any of the pain killers that would be prescribed for post-surgery I made up a pot of the tea the night before.

After my wife got me home and put me to bed she brought in a cup of the tea. I must tell you that the tea has a very strong flavor and will most likely be unpleasant to most people. I personally did not care. I drank the tea and laid back to relax. After about twenty minutes my wife came back to check on me to see if I was in any pain. The mild narcotic properties of the tea not only kept the pain away but made me very happy with a tendency to giggle. For the next few days all I used for a pain killer was a cup of the tea two or three times a day for a few days. I also healed very quickly with no dry sockets from the removal.

It can also be used as a tincture or in capsule form.

DOSAGE: As a tea: 1 cup full as needed for pain. As capsules two to three capsules as needed. As a tincture 2 to four dropperfuls as needed for pain.

Cramp bark and Valerian:

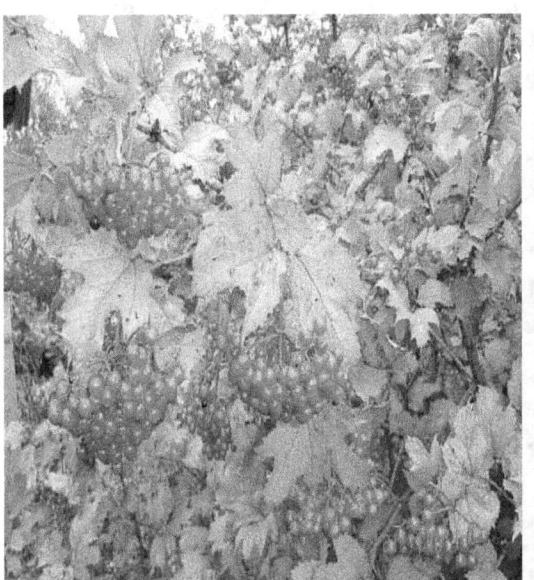 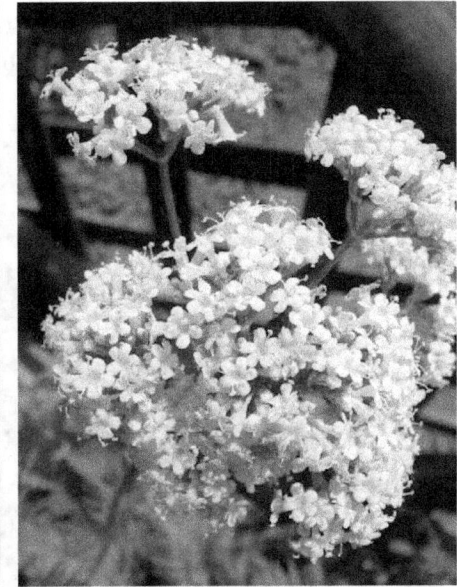

Crampbark and Valerian

This is a wonderful combination we have put together as a mixture of a muscle relaxer and a pain killer. **Cramp bark** (Viburnum opulus) has been used historically by the Native Americans for hundreds of years as a muscle relaxer, especially by women for menstrual cramps. I sprained my back years ago and it was a very effective muscle relaxer.

Valerian (Valeriana officinalis) is well known in the holistic community for it's superb ability for killing pain and for its effect as a tranquilizer and nervine, particularly for those people suffering from nervous over strain. Valerian has been shown to encourage sleep, improve sleep quality and reduce blood pressure. It is also used internally in the treatment of painful menstruation, cramps, hypertension, irritable bowel syndrome etc.

The two herbs are best used as a tincture for faster action. We combine an equal amount of each herb and make an alcohol based tincture from it.

DOSAGE: For adults we usually recommend 1 to 2 dropperfuls as needed for pain. You can increase the dosage easily to four dropperfuls as needed but be aware that the higher the dosage the more relaxed you can become and the "loopier". It may not be safe to drive or operate machinery at higher doses.

Willow (Salix alba):

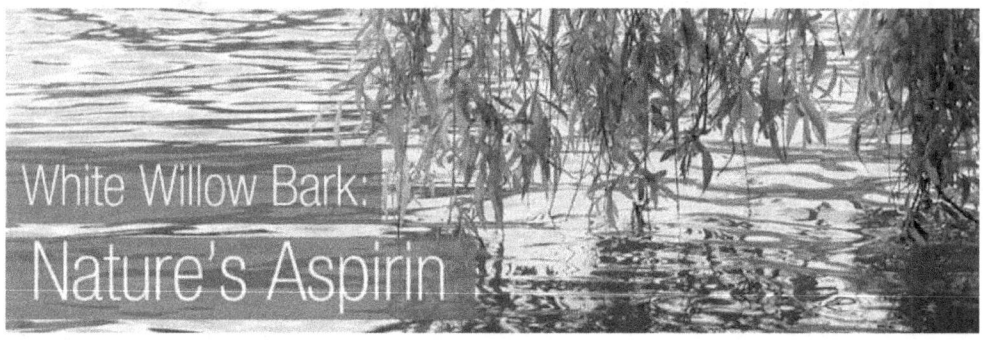

As the picture indicates .. the original source for aspirin. The year was 1899 and Bayer came out with Bayer aspirin. They knew they could not patent a Popular or Willow tree so the worked on extracting what they considered the key ingredient from the plant for relieving pain ... salicin. After purifying it they produced salicylic acid .. aspirin. There was a problem with this extraction though. Left in the original Willow or Poplar bark it is suspended and buffered by hundreds of other chemical constituents. In it's form as aspirin it is not buffered by nature and can eat a hole in your stomach. Not so with Willow.

DOSAGE: We have used it as a tea, capsule or as a tincture. Again, the tincture and tea form are faster acting. The capsule form takes longer to take effect but lasts longer. It is very safe. Use two capsules or dropperfuls or a cup of tea as needed for pain.

CBD:

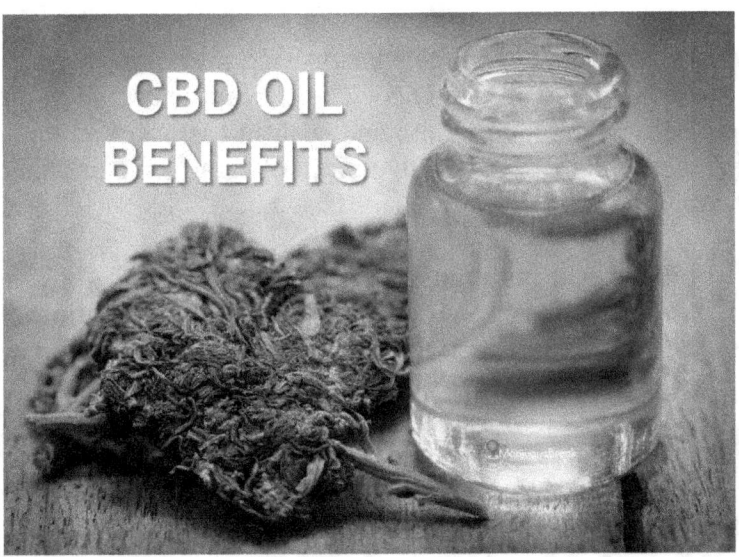

Praised by many and reviled by others, there seems to very little middle ground for the acceptance of this natural remedy. Yes, it does come from Cannabis but we are talking about the form with no THC in it. It does not have any narcotic effects.

We have used it for many years and seen patients who could not take a pharmaceutical drug find relief. Be careful of your supplier of CBD products. Since legalization in many states vendors have come out of the wood work. We prefer to use a company called CV Sciences. They seem to be very consistent in their quality. They are out of Colorado.

DOSAGE: CBD can come in MANY forms. You can get it as capsules, as an oil, salves, sprays, etc. We use it mainly in capsule and salve form. For most folks, they can take one to two of the capsules as needed for pain or to aid in sleeping as needed. The salve is wonderful as a topical application for pain, such as muscle aches.

Castor Oil Packs:

Castor oil packs are age old in their history and are as good today as when they were used hundreds of years ago. The concept is actually quite simple. You take a clean, white cotton cloth and soak in castor oil and place it over the area that is in pain. Cover it with a piece of saran wrap and then a towel. Over the towel you place a heating pad. That's it.

It is able to relieve pain through the use of the castor oil soaking into the skin and getting both the blood and the lymphatic circulation moving. It becomes very cleansing in action and can relieve pain in a matter of minutes.

Benefits of Castor Oil:

1. Positive Influence on the Nervous System.
2. Increases Lymphatic Flow.
3. Works Through the Skin to Reduce Inflammation, Pain and Swelling.
4. Increases Digestive Abilities and Improves Liver Activity.
5. Strengthens the Immune System.

Cayenne Deep Heating:

In an earlier section of this book I discussed Cayenne's ability to be a Rubefacient. This is defined as an herb which can cause a gentle and localized increase in the surface blood flow. This brings along with it more oxygen and nutrients. This will make the area appear red due to the increased blood flow. All of this aids in the healing process which helps diminish pain.

It is well known that a deep heating salve soothes painful and tired muscles. Rather than make our own we generally use Dr. Christopher's Heat ointment.

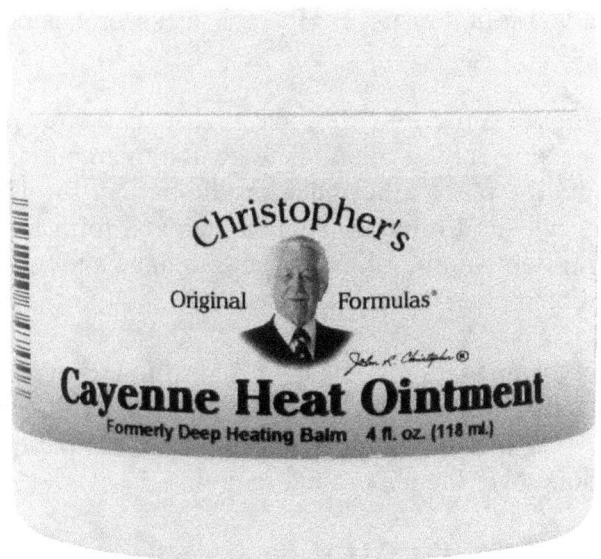

Dr. Christoper's Heat Ointment

Ingredients: Cayenne Pepper (40,000 H.U.), Virgin Olive Oil, Oil of Wintergreen, Menthol Crystals & other pure essential oils as fragrances & Beeswax.

Cold/Hot Packs:

Finally, an oldie but goodie, cold and hot packs. Applying ice or heat can provide relief from injuries, aches, and pains. Ice works for injuries because it narrows your blood vessels, which helps prevent blood from accumulating at the site of injury, which will add to inflammation and swelling while delaying healing. This is also why elevation is helpful, since it limits blood flow to the area to minimize swelling.

For muscle aches and pains, applying a heat pack will help bring blood flow to the area, which promotes healing and soothes pain while increasing flexibility. As blood flow increases, so does the flow of oxygen and nutrients to the area while waste materials are removed. Heat also works well for joint pain or as a pre-workout warm-up. Hot gel packs or heated water bottles work well for this

They are very simple to use and we have seen patients receive great relief from them. The general rule of thumb is to switch them out as each has their own benefits. Initially, place a hot pack on the patient for 12 minutes. The switch to a cold pack for 4 minutes. switch back and forth for as long as the patient feels comfortable doing so. Make sure to have a towel laid down first over the area and then place the packs on top of it.

I have seen cases of appendicitis clear up with the aid of the hot and cold packs being done all night over the area of the appendix. It can also help get the bowels moving during stubborn cases of constipation or a bowel blockage when done over the abdominal region.

HOW TO MAKE THE HOT PACK:
This can be as simple as a hot water bottle or an electric heating pad (some do not care for the EMF coming off of it) or you can fill a sock with rice, sew up the end and heat it in the microwave.

HOW TO MAKE THE COLD PACK:
Again, very simple. Many folks just file a zip-lock bag full of ice.

CHAPTER 10
A SAMPLE FIRST-AID KIT

I would like to take some time now to help you figure out how to make your own Holistic, First Aid kit. In this section we will discuss where to buy them or if you choose to, how to make your own from scratch.

10.1 First Aid Kit Supplies

As far as Dr. Christopher's products are concerned, they can be purchased at Dr. Christoper's Herb Shop online. The website is **https://www.drchristophersherbshop.com**. I will place a * next to the product in the kit if it can be purchased from them or another online source.

Below is a list of what we would put into a home, holistic first aid kit. Please feel free to modify this for your own needs.

FIRST AID KIT SUPPLIES:

For pain relief:
*CBD oil/salve or capsules – CV Sciences 855-758-7223
Cramp bark and Valerian Tincture.
*Willow tincture or capsules – Dr. Christopher's Herb Shop. - 801-489-4500
*Cayenne Heat Ointment - Dr. Christopher's Herb Shop. - 801-489-4500
Aloe Vera gel.

For treating and preventing infection:
Herbadyne
*Garlic oil - Dr. Christopher's Herb Shop. - 801-489-4500
*Infection Formula - Dr. Christopher's Herb Shop. - 801-489-4500

Eye Injuries:
*Herbal Eyebright - Dr. Christopher's Herb Shop. - 801-489-4500

For wound healing:

Green Salve
Comfrey paste ingredients.
*Comfrey root powder - Dr. Christopher's Herb Shop. - 801-489-4500
Raw honey
*Wheatgerm oil - Dr. Christopher's Herb Shop. - 801-489-4500
*Dr. Christopher's Ear and Nerve - Dr. Christopher's Herb Shop. - 801-489-4500
*Dr. Christopher's Complete Tissue and Bone (B, F and C) capsules and salve. Dr. Christopher's Herb Shop. - 801-489-4500

For bleeding/heart attack/strokes/shock:
*Cayenne Tincture - Dr. Christopher's Herb Shop. - 801-489-4500

For poisoning:
*Plantain Tincture - Dr. Christopher's Herb Shop. - 801-489-4500
Activated charcoal

For nausea:
Ginger – As an herb for tea or capsules or drink.

For allergies and allergy related shock:
*Dr. Christopher's Kid-e-Soothe - Dr. Christopher's Herb Shop. - 801-489-4500
*Stinging Nettle tincture – The herb itself can be bought at - Dr. Christopher's Herb Shop. - 801-489-4500. The you can make your own tincture.

Magnifying glass for checking out splinters, ticks, etc.
Tick remover.
Bandages of various sizes.
Gauze pads of various sizes.
Hot water bottle or a heating pad.
Cold pack ready made or a zip-lock bag.
Pack of butterfly bandages.
Ace bandages.
Finger splint.
1 adhesive cloth tape (10 yards x 1 inch)
2 absorbent compress dressings (5 x 9 inches)

Tweezers
2 pairs of non-latex gloves.
Clean cotton cloth.
Bulb syringe.

10.2 How to make your own medications

While it may be convenient to purchase your holistic medications, I feel it is important that we each know how to make our own in a pinch. You can also save a LOT of money should you decide to make your own.

Several of these instructions have already been detailed in this book but I wanted to give you an easy look up for them in one place.

Making a tincture:
The rule of thumb for most tinctures uses a 4:1 ratio of the medium to the herbs. The medium is usually 100 proof vodka as it is 50% water and 50% alcohol. This is the best of both worlds as some herbs require water and some alcohol to be extracted.

For example, if you are going to have 8 ounces of alcohol than you would use 2 ounces of herbs. The herbs can be cut or powdered but powdered can be harder to filter out later in the process.

Place the herbs in the jar and pour in the vodka. Seal and write on it the date you started it. Shake well.

Store in a cool, dark place for two weeks, making sure to walk by at least once a day and shake vigorously.

Drain the tincture though cheesecloth to remove the herbs from the liquid.

Pour the strained tincture into smaller, colored bottles and cap. Be sure to label the bottles. The tincture will keep indefinitely in a cool area.

This formula works well on most herbs, certainly all of those mentioned in this book, including Stinging nettle, Cayenne, Plantain and such.

Making a fomentation:

A fomentation is a cloth soaked in a strong tea and placed over the area of concern. Make a tea out of the herb using 1 teaspoon of the herb to a cup of distilled water or a tablespoon to a pint. Boil the water and not the herb. Let the water boil and when rolling, take off the burner and put the herb in the water, cover and let steep for 20 to 25 minutes or more. Soak the white cotton cloth in it and then place over the area. Cover with saran wrap to keep the moisture and heat in. Leave on for 25 minutes and repeat as often during the day as needed.

Making a Poultice:

A poultice is a wrap made from the actual plant material. Take the plant and tear or break up and put in a pan with distilled water. Put on low simmer for about 25 to 30 minutes. Take the plant materiel out along with some of the water and place on a piece of white, cotton cloth or flannel. Wrap the affected area with the plant in direct contact with the skin and wrap an ace bandage on it to keep it in place. It can be kept on overnight and changed the next day as needed.

Making an infusion (a tea):

An infusion is simply a tea from the flowers, leaves or stems of a plant. Make a tea out of the herb using 1 teaspoon of the herb to a cup of distilled water or a tablespoon to a pint. Boil the water and not the herb. Let the water boil and when rolling, take off the burner and put the herb in the water, cover and let steep for 20 to 25 minutes or more.

Making onion cough syrup:

Take white or yellow onion and chop it up and place into a sauce pan. Cover with raw honey and simmer over low heat for about 25 to 30 minutes. Strain and use the honey as a teaspoon to a tablespoon as needed for coughs.

Making an onion poultice:

To make the poultice, take a white or yellow onion and chop it up thoroughly. Place in the oven at about 250 to 300 degrees for about twenty minutes. You will know when it is done as the pieces are just starting to get "slimy". Now take them out and let them cool enough where they will not damage the skin and place over the chest while the patient is lying down. If this is for a baby then please make sure to rub some olive oil on the skin first to protect it as they are more sensitive than older children or adults.

Making a castor oil pack:

To do this soak a white cotton cloth in castor oil and place it over the skin of the area affected. Now cover the cloth with a saran wrap and then place a towel over the wrap. Now place a heating pad over the towel Do this as many times a day as you can, at least twice a day.

Making an Herbadyne tincture:

Ingredients are 2 ounces of powdered Myrrh, one ounce powdered Golden seal, ½ ounce of powdered cayenne and one quart of 100 proof vodka.

Combine all of the herbs and alcohol in a glass jar, cap tightly and keep it in a cool, shaded area for 14 days. Shake at least once each day. Strain and keep the alcohol in a dark bottle and store in a cool place.

Making a salve:

While this is actually pretty easy, it can take a little practice getting the correct amount of bees wax at the end. Too little and the salve is watery and too much and you might as well be using a rock. Let's give this a try.

You will need the following ingredients:

The herb (Lets try Chickweed for now as a nice skin soother)
Cold pressed, extra virgin, organic Olive oil.
Beeswax.

Place the cut up herb (Chickweed for example) in the pan and cover about an inch over with the Olive oil. Turn the heat on low and let simmer for about 20 minutes. Cover. Try not to let it boil. Check now and then.

After about twenty minutes turn off the heat and move the pan to a burner that is off and cool. Let sit with the cover on it for about 1 hour or more, until it has cooled enough for you to be able to safely strain it. Then strain the oil through a white, cotton cloth or cheese cloth into a bowl.

Clean the previous pan and then put the oil back into it. Turn the heat on to a low setting, careful not to boil. You will need to frequently stir so as not to burn the oil. When the oil is hot, being to CAREFULLY add a little bit of bees wax to the oil and let it melt. Now comes the tricky part. You need to test each time to make sure if you have enough bees wax in the mixture.

To test it, have ready a little saucer or cup with some water in it. Take a little spoonful of the oil and drop into the water. If it remains an oil after cooling than add more bees wax to the hot oil. If it turns to wax then you are done!

Before it has completely cooled, pour in jars and place in the fridge to store. You want it in the fridge relatively soon or it may start to separate. Your done. In a cool, dark place it can last a year at a good potency.

PART THREE – A HOLISTIC APPROACH TO CURING LYME DISEASE

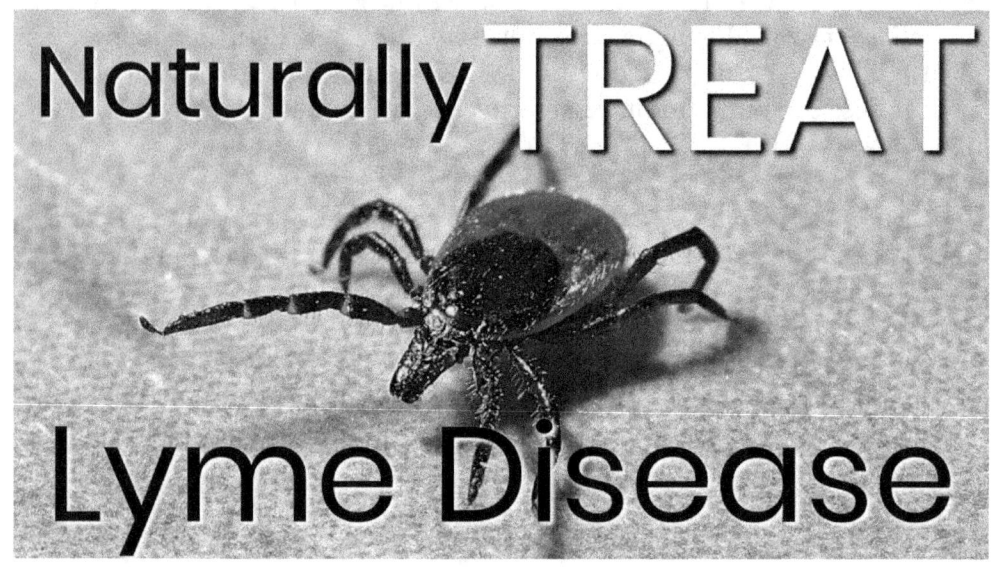

CHAPTER 11

Introduction

The purpose of this book is to offer an alternative treatment for both acute and chronic Lyme disease. To date there are currently 300,000 new cases of Lyme reported in the United States each year. That is six times the reported new cases of HIV. It is the new pandemic of this century. Sadly, most doctors today are either not Lyme-literate or prefer to choose the conventional approach to treatment which is simply symptomatic with high doses of antibiotics. This method has been proven to offer no cure for this disorder and in the end bankrupts most patients. This book will explain in detail the etiology of Lyme, current accepted conventional protocols, along with a treatment plan I have been using in practice for over 20 years. I will also be discussing successful case histories where patients were cured and remain so to this day.

For the past twenty years of practice, from top to bottom, I have treated everything from boo-boo toes to brain cancer. The past seven years we have run one of the largest Traditional Naturopathic medical centers in California called Tree Of Life Holistic Wellness Center. Using holistic, Naturopathic protocols we have seen amazing success in working with issues such as cancer, auto-immune, including as M.S., Lupus, and such. But of all the disorders that have come through our door at the clinic, Lyme would rate as the most difficult and stubborn, and devastating I have witnessed. Another doctor I know of stated once that Lyme was more difficult to treat than cancer. There is some truth to that statement. The Borrelia bacteria, from my perspective, is the most evolved, advanced I have come across. It has an amazing ability to trick the human immune system. If attacked, it will often change the outer protein shell to defeat the antibiotic or it may go into a "cyst" stage and "go to sleep" until the time when the body is weak and ready for another round of attacks.

For years I treated patients, often relying on their previous diagnosis. They would come in with "confirmed" diagnosis for Lupus, Multiple Sclerosis, Rheumatoid Arthritis, Fibromyalgia, Chronic Fatigue Syndrome, etc. I would begin a holistic set of treatments aimed at eliminating the disorders. While they would often find some improvement in their symptoms, the condition itself would persist, sometimes for months or years. Occasionally, they would appear cured, no longer symptomatic. They would leave the clinic happy and looking forward to a healthier life.

Sadly, within months they would return to the clinic as the "old" problem returned. This would often mystify me as I knew from past experience what I had prescribed would work every time for issues such as they presented. I knew in my heart that this should have worked, even in somewhat resistant patients, those who have issues following a protocol.

During this period of time I had begun studying and training in the protocols involving the diagnosis and treatment of Lyme Disease. I began to become suspicious that the original diagnosis from the previous doctors may not have been correct. I started asking patients if we could run a series of tests recommended by Dr. Burrascano, sometimes at a cost to the clinic. We were beginning to suspect there was more going on and when a patient could not afford it and had already spent a great deal of money within the medical system, we would cover the cost of the tests as we were not sure this was actually Lyme.

As it turned out, in so many of the cases, they had been misdiagnosed. It was not unusual for the patients to begin to cry, not from sorrow but joy at finally receiving an actual, correct diagnosis. I applied what I had learned about the manner with which this bacteria attacks the immune system, started treating the co-infections so often present, and we began to see positive, significant results.

Within this book, I will go over the protocols I have used over the years as well as actual case histories of just a few of our success stories. I will compare the success of conventional protocols versus those developed by the holistic community. There is indeed a place for both of us in the medical world as we each contribute to medical wisdom. This will also be the first book in a series detailing the natural, healing protocols for a wide variety of conditions, such as hypertension, diabetes, auto-immune and such. We hope you find this book helpful and please feel free to send me your success stories or personal observations you have experienced in coping with Lyme disease. The clinic's email is clinic@treeoflifehwc.com.

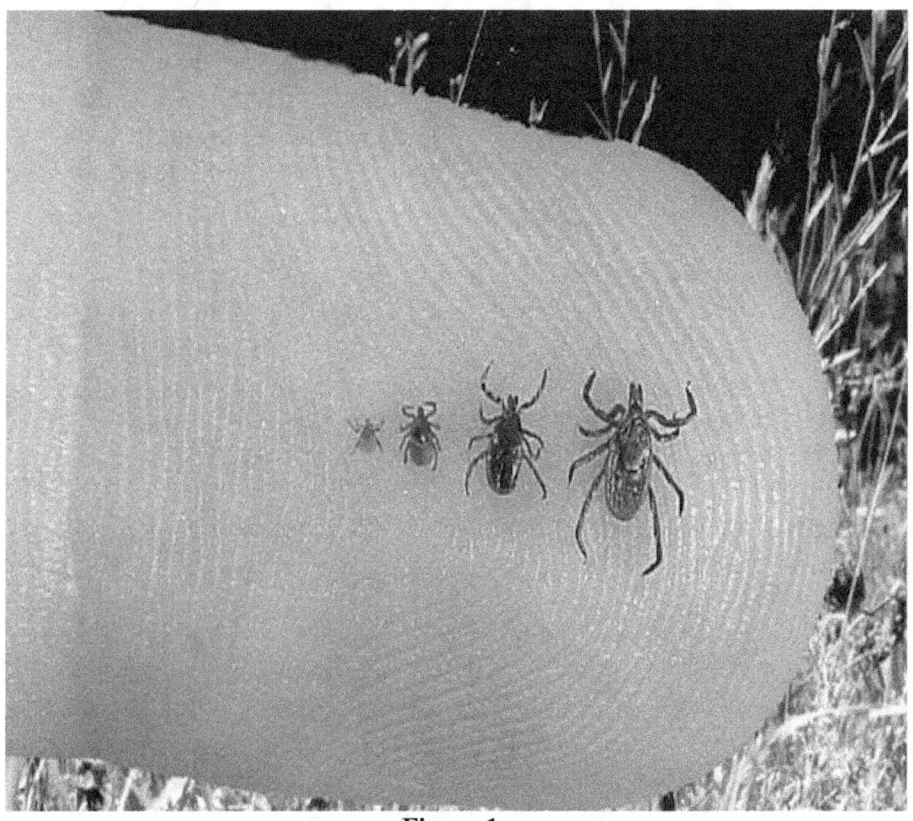

Figure 1

The stages of deer tick growth. Only stages 1 and 4 can transmit the bacteria.

11.1 What is Lyme Disease

In the 1960s and 1970s, something was very wrong in Connecticut. In a population of 12,000 living in three contiguous towns: Old Lyme, Lyme, and East Haddam, 39 children were diagnosed with juvenile rheumatoid arthritis and 12 adults were diagnosed with arthritis of unknown cause.
In 1975, frustrated by the lack of answers from their medical community, two mothers became patient advocates, gathering information from residents that they passed on to the Connecticut State Department of Health and the Yale School of Medicine.

In 1982, the agent responsible for Lyme disease was discovered by Willy Burgdorfer, who isolated spirochetes belonging to the genus Borrelia from the mid-guts of ticks infecting deer, other wild animals, and dogs. Spirochetes are spiral-shaped bacteria that have been identified as early as 30,000 BC. The causative organism was named Borrelia burgdorferi (Bb), after its discoverer.

Following is a quote from JOSEPH J. BURRASCANO JR., M.D. as one of the best definitions for Lyme:

"I take a broad view of what Lyme Disease actually is. Traditionally, Lyme is defined an infectious illness caused by the spirochete, Borrelia burgdorferi (Bb). While this is certainly technically correct, clinically the illness often is much more than that, especially in the disseminated and chronic forms.

Instead, I think of Lyme as the illness that results from the bite of an infected tick. This includes infection not only with B. burgdorferi, but the many co-infections that may also result. Furthermore, in the chronic form of Lyme, other factors can take on an ever more significant role- immune dysfunction, opportunistic infections, coinfections, biological toxins, metabolic and hormonal imbalances, deconditioning, etc. I will refer to infection with B. burgdorferi as "Lyme Borreliosis" (LB), and use the designation "Lyme" and "Lyme Disease" to refer to the more broad definition I described above."

The vast majority of Lyme cases that I have treated over 19 years of practice fits well with the above definition. It is also correct to define it within the parameters of the secondary or co-infections. There have been cases when it was difficult to isolate the B. burgdorferi and yet the tests were clearly positive for such infections as the Babesia bacteria, a common secondary infection associated with Lyme.

Lyme on the march

Cases of Lyme disease have spread across the US as warmer winters encourage the ticks that carry it to move into new areas

● 2001 ● 2005 ● 2010 ● 2015

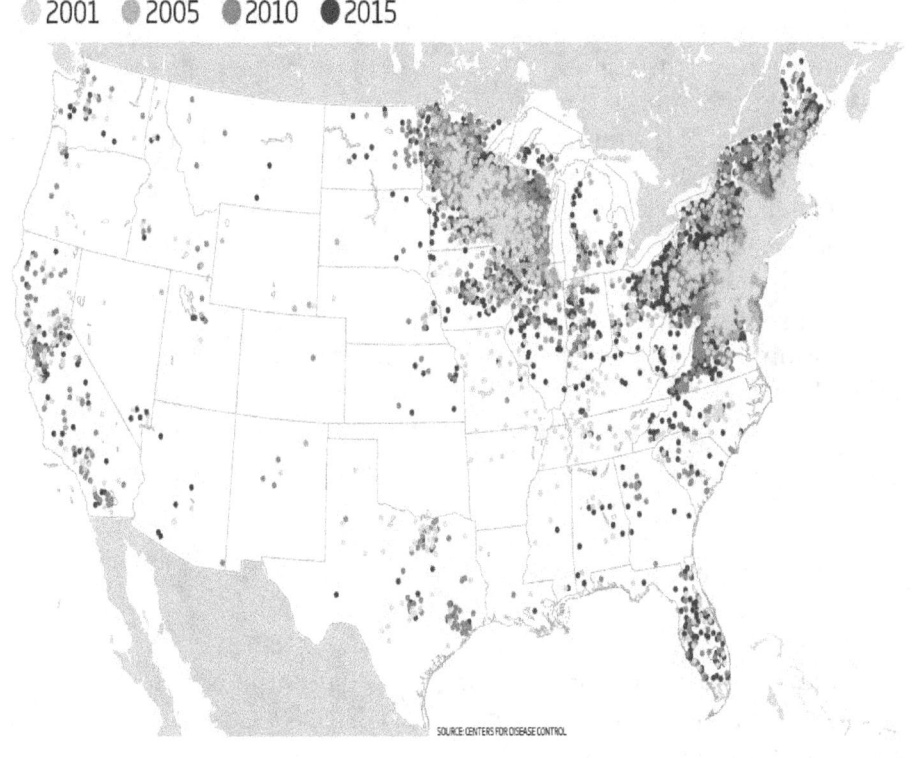

Figure 2.

11.2 Common Symptoms

Unfortunately, this disease is one of the great mimickers as it can appear as dozens of others conditions and is therefore routinely misdiagnosed. Following is a list of symptoms:

Head, Face, Neck
- Unexplained hair loss
- Headache, mild or severe, seizures
- Pressure in head, white matter lesions in brain (MRI)
- Twitching of facial or other muscles
- Facial paralysis (Bell's Palsy, Horner's syndrome)
- Tingling of nose, (tip of) tongue, cheek or facial flushing
- Stiff or painful neck
- Jaw pain or stiffness
- Dental problems
- Sore throat, clearing throat a lot, phlegm (flem), hoarseness, runny nose

Eyes/Vision
- Double or blurry vision
- Increased floating spots
- Pain in eyes, or swelling around eyes
- Oversensitivity to light
- Flashing lights, peripheral waves or phantom images in corner of eyes

Ears/Hearing
- Decreased hearing in one or both ears, plugged ears
- Buzzing in ears
- Pain in ears, over-sensitivity to sounds
- Ringing in one or both ears

Digestive and Excretory Systems
- Diarrhea
- Constipation
- Irritable bladder (trouble starting, stopping) or interstitial cystitis
- Upset stomach (nausea or pain) or GERD (gastroesophageal reflux disease)

Musculoskeletal System
- Bone pain, joint pain or swelling, carpal tunnel syndrome
- Stiffness of joints, back, neck, tennis elbow
- Muscle pain or cramps, (Fibromyalgia)

Respiratory and Circulatory Systems

- Shortness of breath, can't get full/satisfying breath, cough
- Chest pain or rib soreness
- Night sweats or unexplained chills
- Heart palpitations or extra beats
- Endocarditis, heart blockage

Neurologic System
- Tremors or unexplained shaking
- Burning or stabbing sensations in the body
- Fatigue, Chronic Fatigue Syndrome, weakness, peripheral neuropathy or partial paralysis
- Pressure in the head
- Numbness in body, tingling, pinpricks
- Poor balance, dizziness, difficulty walking
- Increased motion sickness
- Light-headedness, wooziness

Psychological Well-being
- Mood swings, irritability, bi-polar disorder
- Unusual depression
- Disorientation (getting or feeling lost)
- Feeling as if you are losing your mind
- Over-emotional reactions, crying easily
- Too much sleep, or insomnia
- Difficulty falling or staying asleep
- Narcolepsy, sleep apnea
- Panic attacks, anxiety

Mental Capability
- Memory loss (short or long term)
- Confusion, difficulty thinking
- Difficulty with concentration or reading
- Going to the wrong place
- Speech difficulty (slurred or slow)
- Difficulty finding commonly used words
- Stammering speech
- Forgetting how to perform simple tasks

Reproduction and Sexuality
- Loss of sex drive
- Sexual dysfunction
- Unexplained menstrual pain, irregularity

- Unexplained breast pain, discharge
- Testicular or pelvic pain

General Well-being
- Phantom smells
- Unexplained weight gain or loss
- Extreme fatigue
- Swollen glands or lymph nodes
- Unexplained fevers (high or low grade)
- Continual infections (sinus, kidney, eye, etc.)
- Symptoms seem to change, come and go
- Pain migrates (moves) to different body parts
- Early on, experienced a "flu-like" illness, after which you have not since felt well
- Low body temperature
- Allergies or chemical sensitivities
- Increased effect from alcohol and possible worse hangover

Figure 3

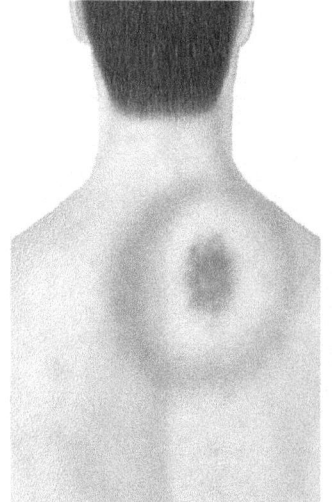
"Classic" erythema migrans rash

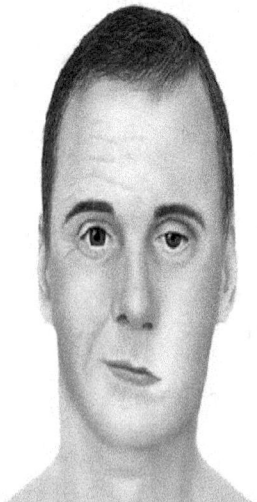
Facial palsy

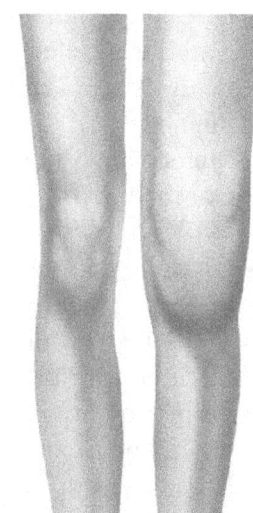
Swollen knee

11.3 A history of misdiagnosis and misinformation

As can be seen from the above list, Lyme is still one of the most misdiagnosed illnesses, hence the reason for both Lyme and Syphilis can be called The Great Imitator.

Patients with Lyme disease have been incorrectly diagnosed with: multiple sclerosis (MS), fibromyalgia, chronic fatigue syndrome, autoimmune diseases including lupus and rheumatoid arthritis [1-7], polymyalgia rheumatica, thyroid disease and psychiatric disorders, among others.

Fatigue, insomnia, and myalgias are seen in both Fibromyalgia and Lyme disease. Chronic Fatigue Syndrome symptoms are often seen in Lyme disease patients and include severe fatigue, impaired memory and concentration, sleep disturbance, myalgias, and arthralgias.

Steere et al. described Lyme disease cases that were misdiagnosed as Juvenile Rheumatoid Arthritis (JRA). [8]

Nowakowski and Feder reported cases misdiagnosed as cellulitis. [9,10]
Plotkin described a 39-year-old male with a retropopliteal rash that progressed, within three weeks to Lyme disease, with a loss of consciousness and a complete heart block that required insertion of a transvenous cardiac pacemaker. [11]
Lyme disease has been mistaken for multiple sclerosis (MS). [12,13] In fact, one author estimated that 5% – 10% of patients presumed to have MS suffered from other conditions including Lyme disease. [14]

Three cases of neuroborreliosis were initially misdiagnosed as anterior ischemic optic neuropathy caused by giant cell arteritis. Neuropsychiatric presentations, including depression, anxiety and rage, have been identified in both acute and chronic Lyme disease cases. [15]

Lyme disease has also been mistaken for polymyalgia rheumatica [16,17], sports related injuries [18], and common medical conditions such as sinusitis, Epstein-Barr syndrome, rotator cuff tear, meniscus tear, edema, cellulitis, and pericarditis. [19].

Other misdiagnosis include:
Flu, Spider Bite, Allergic Hives,
Fibromyalgia, Multiple Sclerosis,
Hypochondria, Adolescent belligerence
Depression, Neurosis
Lupus
Other autoimmune & neurodegenerative
diseases (Alzheimer's & Dementia)

Figure 4

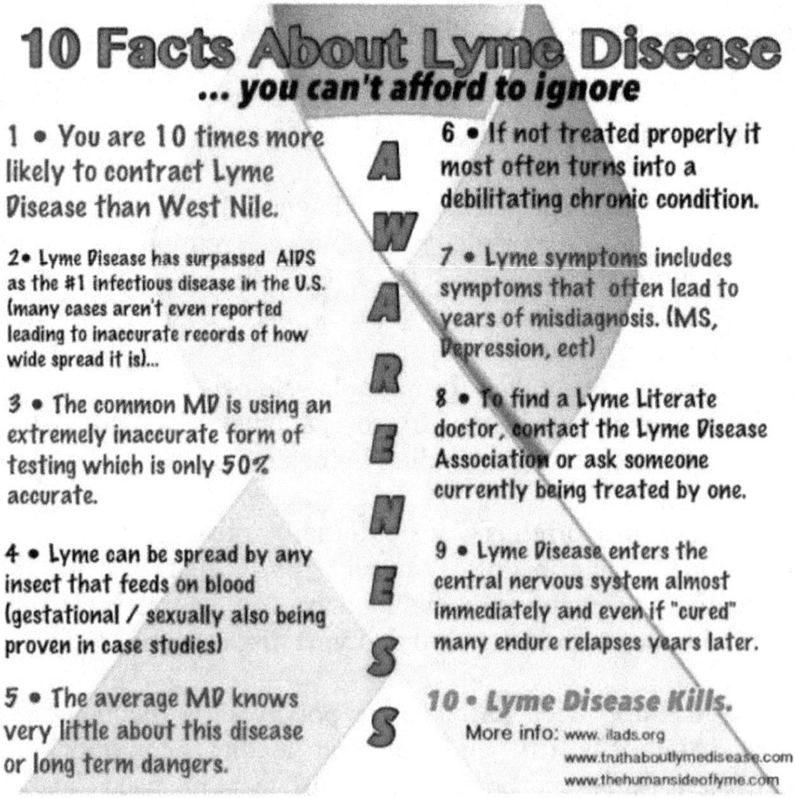

10 Facts About Lyme Disease
... you can't afford to ignore

1 • You are 10 times more likely to contract Lyme Disease than West Nile.

2 • Lyme Disease has surpassed AIDS as the #1 infectious disease in the U.S. (many cases aren't even reported leading to inaccurate records of how wide spread it is)...

3 • The common MD is using an extremely inaccurate form of testing which is only 50% accurate.

4 • Lyme can be spread by any insect that feeds on blood (gestational / sexually also being proven in case studies)

5 • The average MD knows very little about this disease or long term dangers.

6 • If not treated properly it most often turns into a debilitating chronic condition.

7 • Lyme symptoms includes symptoms that often lead to years of misdiagnosis. (MS, Depression, ect)

8 • To find a Lyme Literate doctor, contact the Lyme Disease Association or ask someone currently being treated by one.

9 • Lyme Disease enters the central nervous system almost immediately and even if "cured" many endure relapses years later.

10 • Lyme Disease Kills.

More info: www.ilads.org
www.truthaboutlymedisease.com
www.thehumansideoflyme.com

AWARENESS

11.4 Current methods of diagnosis

The variable signs and symptoms of Lyme disease are nonspecific and often are found in other conditions, so diagnosis can be difficult. What's more, the ticks that transmit Lyme disease also can spread other diseases at the same time.

If you don't have the characteristic Lyme disease rash, your doctor might ask about your medical history, including whether you've been outdoors in the summer where Lyme disease is common, and do a physical exam.

Lab tests to identify antibodies to the bacteria can help confirm the diagnosis. These tests are most reliable a few weeks after an infection, after your body has had time to develop antibodies. They include:

- Enzyme-linked immunosorbent assay (ELISA) test. The test used most often to detect Lyme disease, ELISA detects antibodies to B. burgdorferi. But because it can sometimes provide false-positive results, it's not used as the sole basis for diagnosis. This test might not be positive during the early stage of Lyme disease, but the rash is distinctive enough to make the diagnosis without further testing in people who live in areas infested with ticks that transmit Lyme disease.
- Western blot test. If the ELISA test is positive, this test is usually done to confirm the diagnosis. In this two-step approach, the Western blot detects antibodies to several proteins of B. burgdorferi.
- CD57 Blood Test for Lyme Disease

The Lyme Disease CD57 HNK1 test is used to aid in the diagnosis of Lyme Disease as well as to monitor treatment. Lyme Disease tends to suppress a person's immune system and many people with Lyme have shown a low count for the CD57 Lymphocyte. Typically a CD57 count below 60 is indicative of Lyme Disease. In people being treated for Lyme Disease, monitoring their CD57 count can help determine how well they are responding to treatment. This test can be used as a screening, however not all Lyme people will show a lowered CD57 count and some conditions besides Lyme may lower this count as well. Confirmation with a Western Blot test is recommended.

11.5 Current methods of treatment

Early Lyme Disease

Lyme-literate doctors are likely to recommend more aggressive and longer antibiotic treatment for patients. They may, for instance, treat "high risk" tick bites where the tick came from an endemic area, was attached a long time, and was removed improperly. They may treat a Lyme rash for a longer period of time than the IDSA recommends, to ensure that the disease does not progress. They are unlikely to withhold treatment pending laboratory test results.

Late or Chronic Lyme Disease

Experts agree that the earlier you are treated the better, since early treatment is often successful. Unfortunately, a substantial portion of patients treated with short-term antibiotics continue to have significant symptoms. The quality of life of patients with chronic Lyme disease is similar to that of patients with congestive heart failure. Doctors don't agree about the cause of these ongoing symptoms. The primary cause of this debate is flawed diagnostic testing. There is currently no test that can determine whether a patient has active infection or whether the infection has been eradicated by treatment.

People treated with appropriate antibiotics in the early stages of Lyme disease usually recover rapidly and completely. Antibiotics commonly used for oral treatment include doxycycline, amoxicillin, or cefuroxime axetil. People with certain neurological or cardiac forms of illness may require intravenous treatment with antibiotics such as ceftriaxone or penicillin.
Treatment regimens listed in the following table are for localized (early) Lyme disease. See references below (Hu 2016; Sanchez 2016) for treatment of patients with disseminated (late) Lyme disease. These regimens are guidelines only and may need to be adjusted depending on a person's age, medical history, underlying health conditions, pregnancy status, or allergies.

Age Category	Drug	Dosage	Maximum	Duration, Days
Adults	Doxycycline	100 mg, twice per day orally	N/A	10-21*
	Cefuroxime axetil	500 mg, twice per day orally	N/A	14-21
	Amoxicillin	500 mg, three times per day orally	N/A	14-21
Children	Amoxicillin	50 mg/kg per day orally, divided into 3 doses	500 mg per dose	14-21
	Doxycycline	4 mg/kg per day orally, divided into 2 doses	100 mg per dose	10-21*
	Cefuroxime axetil	30 mg/kg per day orally, divided into 2 doses	500 mg per dose	14-21

Figure 5

Antibiotics are often used to treat Lyme disease. In general, recovery will be quicker and more complete the sooner treatment begins.

Antibiotics

- Oral antibiotics. These are the standard treatment for early-stage Lyme disease. These usually include doxycycline for adults and children older than 8, or amoxicillin or cefuroxime for adults, younger children, and pregnant or breast-feeding women. A 14- to 21-day course of antibiotics is usually recommended, but some studies suggest that courses lasting 10 to 14 days are equally effective.
- Intravenous antibiotics. If the disease involves the central nervous system, your doctor might recommend treatment with an intravenous antibiotic for 14 to 28 days. This is effective in eliminating infection, although it may take you some time to recover from your symptoms. Intravenous antibiotics can cause various side effects, including a lower white blood cell count, mild to severe diarrhea, or colonization or infection with other antibiotic-resistant organisms unrelated to Lyme.

After treatment, a small number of people still have some symptoms, such as muscle aches and fatigue. The cause of these continuing symptoms, known as post-treatment Lyme disease syndrome, is unknown, and treating with more antibiotics doesn't help. Some experts believe that certain people who get Lyme disease are predisposed to develop an autoimmune response that contributes to their symptoms. More research is needed.

Antibiotics can wipe out beneficial intestinal flora, leading to a wide variety of additional health problems. It is important to take probiotics while on antibiotics to maintain a healthy balance of gut bacteria.

Bismacine

The Food and Drug Administration warns against the use of bismacine, an injectable compound prescribed by some alternative medicine practitioners to treat Lyme disease. Bismacine, also known as chromacine, contains high levels of the metal bismuth. Although bismuth is safely used in some oral medications for stomach ulcers, it's not approved for use in injectable form or as a treatment for Lyme disease. Bismacine can cause bismuth poisoning, which may lead to heart and kidney failure.

Orthodox Treatments

Oral antibiotics are the first line of treatment for acute or early disseminated Lyme disease. They are the only proven protocol that effectively treats a Lyme infection. Ì All other treatments are experimental and should not be thought of as replacements for antibiotics. Commonly used antibiotics include: • doxycycline* • amoxicillin (use for children and pregnant women) • cefuroxime axetil • telithromycin

Five to 10 percent of patients treated with doxycycline or amoxicillin (14-30 days) do not respond to treatment (Smith et al 2002). This may be due to co-infections or other unknown factors. * Will also treat ehrlichiosis, STARI, Rocky Mountain spotted fever, human granulocytic anaplasmosis

Intravenous antibiotics are usually used for neurological symptoms and chronic arthralgia associated with PLDS. These include: • ceftriaxone (use five days on, two to three days off to prevent cholecystitis) • benzathine penicillin (can be administered intramuscular or intravenous) • cefotaxime • doxycycline

Oral antibiotics are usually administered for two to four weeks. Some Lyme specialists continue medication at least four to six weeks and combine two to three different types of antibiotics in a protocol for persistent Lyme disease. Intravenous antibiotics are administered at least four to six months, even though there are no studies confirming the effectiveness of this therapy beyond a six week time frame. The common side effects associated with oral antibiotics include nausea, diarrhea, sun sensitivity, vaginal yeast infections, rash, glossitis, and abdominal pain. The use of probiotics with fructo-oligosaccharides (FOS) during antibiotic treatment can reduce many of the digestive yeast overgrowth and antibiotic related colitis (Clostridium difficile) side effects associated with antibiotic use. Many of the IV antibiotics require a central line, as they are caustic and they frequently cause a Jarisch Herxheimer-like reaction in patients.

A review by Warshafsky et al suggests that if a prophylactic antibiotic is given within 72 hours of a tick bite, it is effective for preventing transmission of Lyme disease (Warshafsky et al 2010). In the original study (Nadelman 2001) a single 200-mg dose of doxycycline prevented patients from developing Lyme disease 87 percent of the time compared to placebo. Readers should be aware that even with the placebo, transmission rates were surprisingly low. Most Lyme specialists would strongly advise against using this type of abrogated therapy.

In persistent Lyme disease, the use of steroids and other immunosuppressive medications should be absolutely avoided as they contribute to the progression of this illness and will likely cause treatment failure. Lack of sleep, alcohol use (except for small amounts in tinctures), cigarette smoking, and nutrient deficiencies can also contribute to poor patient response.

Why Antibiotics May Not Work for Lyme Disease
- Borrelia burgdorferi, the bacteria that causes Lyme disease, has a corkscrew shape that allows it to bore deep into tissues and cartilage (including the brain and nervous system), safely out of reach of most antibiotics.
- Borrelia burgdorferi can give up its corkscrew shape and convert to a form that is able to live inside cells ("intracellular") where again, antibiotics have less reach.
- Borrelia burgdorferi, along with other similar microbes, can form dormant cysts that are completely resistant to antibiotics; the harder you hit it, the more resistant it becomes.
- Borrelia burgdorferi is usually accompanied and aided by co-infections of other stealth microbes that also live inside cells.

Antibiotic resistance occurs at a high rate with these types of microbes. An antibiotic is one single chemical substance. Bacteria, such as Borrelia (and also its co-infections), respond slowly to antibiotics and have more time to develop resistance to the antibiotic. In other words, the longer they can hang on, the more likely they are to become completely antibiotic resistant. Using multiple antibiotics at once seems to accelerate this process and alternating antibiotics doesn't seem to help. Resistant bacteria become even more entrenched.

Antibiotics destroy the normal flora (friendly bacteria) in the gut and skin, causing bacterial imbalance and a host of other symptoms in the body. Most importantly, use of antibiotics suppresses immune function, which may present the greatest hurdle to recovery—you cannot get well without optimal immune function.

Borrelia burgdorferi can exist in biofilms, which are protected colonies of microbes that form on a surface (such as plaque on your teeth), but what role this plays in Lyme disease is controversial. The symptom profile of Lyme disease suggests that it is not a biofilm disease and that biofilms are not a big factor in overcoming Lyme.

CHAPTER 12

Holistic Protocols

Natural treatment options for Lyme disease are often more effective than antibiotics and prescription medication. Tweaking the daily diet as well as supplementing one's daily routine often relieve the symptoms of Lyme disease and naturally cure the condition. Small changes like exercising, taking probiotics and adding herbs to a daily routine destroys Lyme bacteria in the body and reduces symptoms.

Your Gut and Your immune System

Chronic infection is an underlying factor in most chronic illnesses. Our sugar-laden diet, GMO foods that kill beneficial bacteria, antibiotics, other antibacterial products, and many of the chemicals in our food supply deplete our beneficial bacteria, which wreaks havoc on our immune systems. This sets the stage for systemic, chronic fungal infections and parasites to multiply, permeate the gut, enter the body's bloodstream, and spread infection throughout the body.

Conventional doctors are very bad at finding and diagnosing parasitical and fungal infections that cannot easily be seen on the surface of the body. The average person is dealing with Candida overgrowth at the very least (the most common fungal infection in our bodies) due to the aforementioned modern diet and lifestyle.
Obviously, to treat a difficult bacterial infection such as Lyme (or whatever combination of bacteria, viruses, and parasites causing Lyme symptoms) the immune system needs to be as strong as possible. The immune system is only as healthy as the gut. The body's intestinal tract mirrors the body's health and dictates the power of the immune system. Step one is to balance the gut flora and eliminate most of the harmful pathogens in the body.

Diet

A healthy diet relies on a foundation of on raw, fresh, organic (when possible), whole foods and herbs. A vegan diet has proven over an over again as the most optimal diet for supplying the body the micro-nutrients need to support the immune system. Salads are one of the best ways to do this. Not your typical iceberg lettuce salads with a few carrots shreds and some ranch dressing, but a salad with a wide variety of at least 10 different vegetables along with fresh garlic, turmeric, ginger, unrefined sea salt, and healthy fats. It is the best way to get a wide array of the best nutrients that will repair the gut and rebuild the body's immune system. Don't underestimate this; a large salad every day, done right, will do more for the body than any supplement regimen, and when followed long enough, the right diet with these kinds of daily salads can completely heal the body from disease, in most cases. But the right supplement protocol can radically speed things up and is often necessary for the very ill.

A perfect diet would not be complete without lots of clean drinking water. For detoxification, cranberry Stevia lemonade is very good for rejuvenating the kidneys, cleaning the liver, purifying blood, and flushing out the whole system. For most people, a gallon a day will yield remarkable results, but for smaller people, or those who have rare conditions that make this dangerous, use common sense and don't ever drink too much water (or any fluid). And for everyone else, a gallon of cranberry lemonade every day will have amazing benefits, second only to salads and cutting out other junk food, but again, use common sense. Drinking that much water in a very short period of time can kill people, believe it or not.

Lifestyle Remedies for Tick-Borne Illness
If caught early enough, Lyme disease can typically be treated using several lifestyle remedies. Regular exercise augments the amount of oxygen in the body and blood, which acts to destroy the Lyme bacteria in the blood. Additionally, probiotics taken daily boosts the number of good bacteria in the gut, supplementing the immune system.

Herbal Treatment for Lyme

Certain herbs have also been shown to suppress microbial threats like Lyme disease. Andrographis, cat's claw and sarsaparilla constitute three of the most important Lyme disease treatment options. These herbs effectively suppress Lyme bacteria with limited side effects or reactions.

Andrographis

An antiviral and antibacterial herb, andrographis has proven to also have patristic properties. Often used in treatment for common viral illnesses, this herb delivers a variety

of healing properties. Regular dosing of this herb delivers liver protection, immune enhancement and cardiovascular benefits, making it a good addition to a Lyme disease fighting regimen.

Cat's Claw

Known for its treatment of microbial conditions, cat's claw is an herb used primarily in treating Lyme disease. The herb offers several healing properties including antiparisitic, anti-inflammatory and antioxidant benefits.

Sarsaparilla

An antibacterial herb, sarsaparilla is particularly effective for treating infection. Additionally, it delivers anti-inflammatory properties and antioxidant benefits. Sarsaparilla is a safe, natural Lyme disease cure.

Early detection is key to successful treatment of Lyme. However, following a strict, natural treatment regimen can offer extensive benefits at any stage of the disease.

Alternatives for Treating Persistent Lyme Disease Syndrome (PLDS)

Many patients with PLDS are highly resistant to treatment. There are several causes for this. First, the Borrelia burgdorferi (Bb) organism can be found in blood and intercellular fluids as well as muscle, nerve, and organ tissue. No single antibiotic is effective for treating infections disseminated in both bodily fluids and various tissues. Secondly, Bb is pleomorphic and can exist in at least two and possibly three forms (Miklossy et al 2008). The L-form, or spheroplast, has no cell wall and is not susceptible to the same types of antibiotics as is the spirochete. A third possible form, a cyst form, is controversial, but may be able to lie dormant during conventional treatment and they cannot be killed by most antibiotics. Metronidazole and tinidazole are recommended (Burrascano 2008).

The following protocol has been used with some success in patients with PLDS that had previously been treated with oral and intravenous antibiotics. Most of these patients were symptom-free as long as they continued intravenous antibiotics, but for various reasons (especially cost) they were unable to continue with that therapy. Of the 150+ patients that I have treated using various incarnations of this protocol (several hundred people under the supervision of other clinicians have also been treated with my protocol), approximately 65 percent are symptom free or have greatly reduced symptoms; 20 percent showed moderate improvement, and 15 percent did not respond. A larger, well-designed study is needed to substantiate these clinical findings.

Herbal Therapy

Lyme Formula #1: Spirolyd Compound™ (by Herbalist & Alchemist) Dosage: 3-4 ml TID. Take for two weeks before adding in the Spirolyd Support™ formula. Patients with gastritis or gastric ulcers should take with food to prevent further GI irritation.

- Sarsaparilla rhizome (Smilax spp.) –traditional syphilis treatment; anti-inflammatory; alterative
- Guaiac resin (Guaiacum officinale) – traditional syphilis treatment; anti-inflammatory; antibacterial
- Stillingia root (Stillingia sylvatica) – traditional syphilis treatment; clears blood heat; alterative
- Andrographis herb (Andrographis paniculata) – clears blood heat (infections); antiamoebic, antibacterial and hepatoprotective

- Prickly ash bark (Zanthoxylum clava-herculis) –antibacterial and antiviral; relieves bone pain and arthralgia; enhances circulation and absorption

Lyme Formula #2: Spirolyd Support™ by Herbalist & Alchemist Dosage: 2-4 ml TID. Take concurrently with Spirolyd Compound™ for two weeks, then discontinue for two weeks, then reintroduce for two weeks. This pattern should be continued throughout treatment.

The rationale for this second formula is that the Borrelia spirochete can become resistant to treatment if the same antibiotic or herb is used. The addition of the second formula is designed to prevent resistance, which supposedly with herbs should not occur, but clinically seems to happen in some cases.
- Houttuynia herb (Houttuynia cordata) – clears blood heat (infections); antibacterial, antiviral and antifungal • Teasel root (Dipsacus asper) – anti-inflammatory; helps relieve arthralgia • Boneset herb (Eupatorium perfoliatum) –diaphoretic, antibacterial and immunostimulant; relieves bone and muscle pain • Isatis root (Isatis indigotica) –antibacterial and antiviral; clears blood heat (infections) • Lomatium root (Lomatium dissectum) –antibacterial, antiviral and antifungal

Note: The herbs alone are not effective to resolve Lyme disease (except for in canines).

Heat Therapy

Daily elevation of core body temperature to 101.5 to 102 degrees Fahrenheit, once per day for 15 minutes, inhibits Borrelia reproduction and enhances effectiveness of the herbal or antibiotic treatment (Reisenger 1996). Take care to hydrate the patient and replace lost minerals, especially calcium, magnesium and zinc.

Saunas, hot tubs, and steam baths are probably the most effective methods for elevating body temperature. If not available, hot baths combined with taking a diaphoretic tea [yarrow (Achillea millefolium), elderflower (Sambucus nigra), ginger (Zingiber officinale)] can be substituted.

Note: Fever therapy alone is not effective to resolve Lyme disease.

These therapies together show greater activity than either one alone. Combining the use of the herbs and elevation of body temperature with antibiotic therapy results in improved outcomes over antibiotics alone or alternative therapies alone.

Other Proposed "Cures" for Lyme Disease

Teasel root (Dipsacus fullonum) – Some herbalists claim to have had success treating Lyme disease with very small doses of the common weedy teasel root. My clinical experience with this herb has confirmed that it is effective for relieving joint pain (Lyme arthralgia), but I have not been able to duplicate their experience in resolving confirmed cases of Lyme disease with my patients. I prefer to use the Asian xu duan (D. asper, D. japonica) as it seems to me to be more effective and less likely to cause nausea and digestive upset.

Spilanthes (Spilanthes acmella) is claimed by some practitioners to have antibacterial activity, especially against spirochetes. I know of no published data to support this claim. The herb does have antibacterial, antifungal, and immunostimulating effects.

Cat's claw bark (Uncaria tomentosa, U. guianensis) – A small study (28 people) was done comparing a tetracyclic oxindole alkaloid- (TOA) free cat's claw product with antibiotic therapy. Reportedly, 85 percent of the cat's claw group (14 people) were seronegative after six months for Bb and had dramatic improvement in their symptoms. The control group treated with antibiotics fared poorly. This study by Cowden, W., Moayad, H., et al, is available as a preliminary report on the Internet (http://www.samento.com.ec/sciencelib/sarticles/Studyshowssamento.htm) and has never been published as far as I can tell. There are many questions about the study's validity. In addition, the whole TOA and pentacyclic oxindole alkaloid (POA) controversy concerning Uncaria is false and based on marketing rather than science. Cat's claw does clear blood heat (infections) and may be of some benefit for treating Lyme disease, but in clinical practice when used by itself it has not produced dramatic improvements in most people that I have treated.

Japanese knotweed root (Polygonum cuspidatum) – Many websites promote this herb as a "cure" for Lyme disease. It is useful for treating Lyme arthralgia (Damp-Heat arthritis) and is a rich source of resveratrol, which is an effective antioxidant and anti-inflammatory. While the root has antibacterial activity and can be a useful part of a Lyme protocol, I do not believe it is a cure for Lyme disease.

Homeopathic ledum (Ledum palustre) is recommended to prevent and treat Lyme disease. It is also widely used in the veterinary community to treat canine and equine cases. While anecdotal stories of Lyme "cures" and improvements abound, there are no studies that I am aware of showing this treatment is effective.

Herbal/Nutritional Protocols for Lyme Disease Symptoms

Muscle and neck pain or spasm

• Ashwagandha root (Withania somnifera) is an adaptogen, antispasmodic and anxiolytic useful for muscle or fibromyalgia pain. • Black cohosh root (Actaea racemosa) is an antispasmodic and analgesic used for muscle pain. Do not use it with hepatotoxic antibiotics. • Blue vervain herb (Verbena hastata) is effective for muscle spasms and facial tics that are exacerbated by stress. Use it with carminatives to prevent nausea. • Siler/Ledebouriella, fang feng root (Saposhnikovia divaricata) is effective for treating Liver Wind muscle spasms or migratory pain. • Gambir, gou teng thorns (Uncaria sinensis) have antispasmodic and analgesic activity and are used to treat spasms, facial and neck pain. • Kava root (Piper methysticum) is an effective muscle antispasmodic, analgesic and anxiolytic. Do not use it with hepatotoxic antibiotics. • Kudzu root (Pueraria lobata) is used to relieve muscle spasms, stiff neck, or sore, achy muscles. • Magnesium, 400-600 mg per day, is effective for treating muscle spasms, restless leg syndrome and facial tics. Take either liquid magnesium or the L-lactate dihydrate form. Topical magnesium gels also seem to be effective. • Skullcap herb (Scutellaria lateriflora) is a nervine for patients who develop nervous tics, tremors, palsies, and spasms under stress. It is also of benefit for headaches where the scalp muscles are sore. • Wood betony herb (Pedicularis spp.) is used for muscles that feel tired, overworked, and sore.

Lyme arthralgia (joint pain)

• Ba ji tian root (Morinda officinalis) is used for knee, ankle, and low back pain. It is also an antidepressant and may have mild adaptogenic effects. • Glucosamine (500 mg-1000 mg) with MSM (500 mg) BID/TID is useful for painful joints and arthritic pain. It has anti-inflammatory activity. • Japanese knotweed root, hu zhang (Polygonum cuspidatum) clears Damp-Heat and WindDamp conditions with blood stasis and pain. It is useful for Lyme arthralgia and contains resveratrol, which is a potent antioxidant and anti-inflammatory. • Huai niu xi root (Achyranthes bidentata) is used in Traditional Chinese Medicine (TCM) for painful tendons, ligaments, and joints. • Solomon's seal root (Polygonatum biflorum) is especially useful for joint, disc, and cartilage pain and injuries. • Teasel root, xu duan (Dipsacus asper) is an effective anti-inflammatory for painful joints, tendons, and ligaments and it significantly helps Lyme arthralgia. • Coix seed, yi yi ren (Coix lachryma-jobi) increases joint mobility, has anti-inflammatory activity and relieves muscle spasms.

General Anti-inflammatories for Lyme arthralgia

• Alpha lipoic acid is useful for Lyme-induced peripheral neuropathy. It also promotes Co-Q-10 absorption and improves antioxidant status (250 mg BID). • Blueberry fruit (Vaccinium spp.) is a nutritive anti-inflammatory which benefits visual and cognitive problems and reduces allergic response. • Boswellia gum (Boswellia serrata) is a warming anti-inflammatory, analgesic and antifungal agent. • Cat's claw bark (Uncaria tomentosa, U. guianensis) is an immunomodulator and cooling antiinflammatory. It heals the gut mucosa and is useful for leaky gut syndrome. • Chai hu root (Bupleurum chinensis) is a cooling anti-inflammatory, hepatoprotective and antibacterial agent. I use it for migratory pain caused by Lyme disease. • EPA/DHA (Omega 3 flax oils) are anti-inflammatory and reduce inflammatory prostaglandin production (4-6 g per day). • Ginger rhizome (Zingiber officinale) is a warming anti-inflammatory and carminative. • Sarsaparilla rhizome (Smilax spp.) is a cooling anti-inflammatory. It binds endotoxins in the gut, enhancing their excretion, and may be useful for promoting excretion of Babesia hemotoxins. • Turmeric rhizome (Curcuma longa) is hepatoprotective, a warming anti-inflammatory, and it heals the gut mucosa. • Yucca root (Yucca spp.) is a cooling anti-inflammatory used for arthritic pain.

Neurological and cognitive symptoms including poor memory, lack of concentration, and confusion • Acetyl-L-carnitine can help improve cognitive function, mood and memory (1500-2000 mg per day). • Bacopa herb (Bacopa monnieri) is an anxiolytic, nootropic, nervine and thyroid stimulant. • Ginkgo standardized extract (Ginkgo biloba) is a cerebral stimulant, antioxidant and it inhibits platelet activating factor (PAF). • Gotu kola herb (Centella asiatica) is a cerebral stimulant, anti-inflammatory and anxiolytic.
  • Holy basil (Ocimum tenuiflorum) is a mild adaptogen, cerebral stimulant, antioxidant, and antibacterial. • Lemon balm herb (Melissa officinalis) is a nervine, antibacterial and carminative. • Rhodiola root (Rhodiola rosea) is a stimulating adaptogen, antidepressant and antioxidant. • Rosemary herb (Rosmarinus officinalis) is a cerebral stimulant, antibacterial and carminative. • St. John's wort flowering herb (Hypericum perforatum) is a nervine, antidepressant and antiinflammatory. It is also used for nerve pain. • Schisandra berry, wu wei zi (Schisandra chinensis) is an adaptogen, nootropic, hepatoprotective agent and antioxidant. It is calming and provides a feeling of alertness and increased focus. • White peony root, bai shao (Paeonia lactiflora) enhances cognitive function, is a nootropic and it relieves brain fog caused by deficient blood.

Bell's palsy • Mullein root (Verbascum thapsus) is specific for facial nerve pain and inflammation. • Prickly ash bark (Zanthoxylum spp.) is a circulatory stimulant and it relieves peripheral nerve pain. • St. John's wort flowering tops (Hypericum perforatum) is useful for nerve pain and inflammation. • Sub-lingual B-12 (methylcobalamin form only) often works in three to seven days to relieve Bell's palsy (1 mg/day). • Sweet melilot herb (Melilotus alba or M. officinalis) is indicated for sharp, stabbing nerve pain.

Lyme insomnia • Biota seed, bai zi ren (Platycladus orientalis) calms disturbed Shen and is useful for treating insomnia, anxiety, fear, night sweats, and cardiac palpitations. • Gambir, gou teng thorns (Uncaria sinensis) are useful for irritability and anxiety inhibiting sleep. • Hops strobiles (Humulus lupulus) are sedative, anxiolytic and analgesic. • Passionflower herb (Passiflora incarnata) is a nervine/sedative, relieves circular thinking, and occipital headaches. • Ye jiao teng stem (Polygonum multiflorum) calms disturbed Shen; use with jujube seed and passionflower for insomnia, anxiety and nightmares. • Jujube seed, suan zao ren (Zizyphus spinosa) calms disturbed Shen and is effective for treating insomnia, nightmares, palpitations, and anxiety.

Lyme anxiety • Bacopa herb (Bacopa monnieri) is an anxiolytic, nootropics and nervine. • Blue vervain herb (Verbena hastata) is an anxiolytic and it helps control muscle spasms and nervous tics. • Chinese Polygala root, yuan zhi (Polygala tenuifolia) is a strong anxiolytic and sedative. • Fresh oat (Avena sativa) is a nervine and mild anxiolytic for people who are emotionally brittle or highly labile. • Motherwort herb (Leonurus cardiaca) is an anxiolytic and nervine, it helps controls cardiac palpitations. • Pulsatilla herb (Anemone patens) is a strong anxiolytic used for panic attacks. It is toxic in overdose.
 • Ye jiao teng stem (Polygonum multiflorum) calms disturbed Shen, use it with jujube seed and passionflower for insomnia, anxiety and nightmares.

Fatigue and HPA axis depletion • American ginseng root (Panax quinquefolius) is a nourishing adaptogen and immune amphoteric. • Ashwagandha root (Withania somnifera) is a calming adaptogen, especially if the patient has hypothyroid function and low hemoglobin. It is also an immune amphoteric. • Asian ginseng root, ren shen (Panax ginseng) is a stimulating adaptogen, anti-inflammatory and immune amphoteric. Red ginseng is most appropriate for people who are cold, deficient and exhausted. • Co-Q-10 (Ubiquinone) enhances energy and oxygenation of tissues (100 mg TID). • Cordyceps fungus, dong chong xia cao (Cordyceps chinensis) nourishing adaptogen, immune amphoteric. It also has hepato- and nephroprotective activity. • Eleuthero root (Eleutherococcus senticosus) is a mild adaptogen, immune amphoteric and antioxidant. • Holy basil herb (Ocimum tenuiflorum) is a mild adaptogen, nootropic and immune amphoteric. • Rhodiola root (Rhodiola rosea) is a stimulating adaptogen, antidepressant, antioxidant and cardiac tonic. • Schisandra berry, wu wei zi

(Schisandra chinensis) is a calming adaptogen, hepatoprotective, antioxidant and immune amphoteric.

Immunodeficiency in persistent Lyme disease: • Astragalus root, huang qi (Astragalus membranaceus) is an immune amphoteric and it has cardioprotective and nephroprotective activity. • Cat's claw bark (Uncaria tomentosa, U. guianensis) is an immune amphoteric and antibacterial agent. • Chaga sclerotium (Inonotus obliquus) is an immunopotentiator. • Maitake mushroom (Grifola frondosa) is an immune amphoteric. • Reishi mushroom, ling zhi (Ganoderma sinensis) is an immune amphoteric and mild calming adaptogen. • Also see adaptogens under Fatigue.

To prevent liver damage due to the use of potentially hepatotoxic antibiotics [tetracycline, cefriaxone, atovaquone (used for babesiosis), minocycline, and high-dose doxycycline]: • Standardized milk thistle seed (Silybum marianum) is hepatoprotective, antioxidant and antiinflammatory. • Schisandra berry, wu wei zi (Schisandra chinensis) is hepatoprotective, antioxidant and antiinflammatory. • Turmeric (Curcuma longa) is hepatoprotective, antioxidant and anti-inflammatory.

Herbs used to help prevent yeast overgrowth from long-term antibiotic use: • Berberine-containing herbs are antifungal, they include goldenseal (Hydrastis canadensis), Chinese coptis (huang lian, Coptis chinensis), Oregon grape root (Mahonia spp.), barberry (Berberis spp.), yellow root (Xanthorhiza simpliccisima). • Cardamom seed (Elettaria cardamomum) is antifungal and inhibits Candida albicans. It is also antibacterial. • Fireweed herb (Epilobium angustifolium) is antifungal and inhibits Candida albicans.
 • Garlic bulb (Allium sativum) is antifungal and inhibits Candida albicans. It also has antibacterial activity. • Spilanthes herb (Spilanthes acmella) is antifungal and inhibits Candida albicans. It also has antibacterial activity. • Probiotics and fermented foods help prevent depletion of normal healthy bowel and vaginal flora and inhibit overgrowth of pathogenic bacteria, fungi and yeast.

12.1 My Protocols to date

In my 20 years of practice I have found a holistic program to be much more effective in treating chronic diseases such as Lyme disease than the currently accepted protocols with conventional medicine. As holistic implies, this utilizes cleansing protocols, dietary, nutrition and lifestyle changes, herbal medicine, exercise, fresh air, etc. I have found if patients consistently follow the program as laid out we have found a very high success rate with the Lyme bacteria undetectable in the blood along with cessation of the collateral damage caused by the original infection. In this section I will layout the protocol, step by step as I have used it in my practice.

TIME LINE:

With most cases, I have seen cures for chronic Lyme normally taking anywhere from nine months to a year, depending on the severity of the case as well as the commitment of the patient. A cure is defined as the following:

a.) No live Borrilis bacteria is detectable in the blood.
b.) The CD57 is 200 and above.
c.) Any sign co-infections is not longer present in the blood.
d.) All previous symptoms of chronic Lyme have been eliminated.
Acute Lyme, meaning the patient has not been infected for any longer than three months, we have seen the above definition of a cure averaging three months.

12.2 CANDIDA CLEANSE:

The first step in my program is to aid the patient in returning the immune system back to a state where it can begin to fight the disease. Since one of the most common disorders affecting the immune system in this country is a candida overgrowth, we start with a cleanse to purge the body of excess of candida and begin to re-establish the micro-flora environment.

Definition of a Candida Overgrowth

The perforated bowel is referred to as Leaky Gut Syndrome. This condition also allows undigested protein to enter the bloodstream. These proteins are foreign to the immune system and are therefore attacked. The immune system remembers these protein invaders and reacts like an allergy each time you consume them. This opens up the possibility of eventually making you allergic to every food you eat.

Since yeast overgrowth can cause symptoms mimicking many diseases, misdiagnosis is common and yeast overgrowth remains undetected allowing it to further colonize, thus creating more side effects and ill health. Many people have suffered for decades going from doctor to doctor, therapy to therapy and eventually being prescribed anti-depressants from doctors who are incapable of a proper diagnosis, so they determine that it is in the head of the patients. This incompetence on the part of modern medicine hopefully leads these unfortunate patients to alternative therapy.

Most alternative therapy focuses on killing off the yeast and providing the body with the pro- biotics. These therapies fail to correct the damaged intestinal tract which allows the yeast condition to return. The following twenty day protocol addresses all aspects of treatment and can permanently eliminate Systemic Yeast Overgrowth and Leaky Gut Syndrome.

First procedure: On the first two days consume two quarts of a decoction of Black Walnut and Pau d' arco (one quart each day). This is made by simmering the herbs in water for twenty minutes at the rate of one tablespoon of the combined herbs (equal parts) per cup of water. An easier alternative would be to take five capsules five times a day of Dr. Christopher's Intestinal Sweep Formula. This procedure will kill off the yeast, which on other programs can make you feel very nauseous. This nauseous feeling is avoided by taking plant-based digestive enzymes in large amounts (triple the stated dosages on the label) and flushing out with Dr. Christopher's Lower Bowel formula during these first two days. NOTES: The Lower Bowel formula can be taken the whole time if needed. You should have 3 bowels movements a day and the amount of Lower Bowel taken is the amount needed to give you 3 bowel movements a day. It is most important during that first procedure so that the body is eliminating the yeast etc. Udo's Choice has plant-based digestive enzymes, which are available at most herb shops.

Second procedure: For the next 14 days, take five capsules five times per day of Dr. Christopher's Soothing Digestion formula, or one tablespoon of slippery elm gruel five times a day. Either of these methods will coat, soothe and heal the lesions in the intestinal wall. (You can continue to take the Intestinal Sweep Formula 2 capsules 3 times a day during this time.)

Third procedure: For the next two days repeat the first procedure.

Fourth procedure: Take copious (triple the stated dosages on the label) amounts of multi-strain Pro- biotics to re-establish the flora. Further aids would be to eat raw sauerkraut, Kim Chi, raw apple cider vinegar, Rejuvelac, or miso in large amounts, which are the exact foods to stay away from if you have leaky gut syndrome, yet they rebuild the flora once the leaky gut is healed. NOTES: Udo's Choice has Pro-biotics, are available at most herb shops. The pro-biotics need to be taken for about a week to rebuild the flora. Note: It is absolutely essential that you do not feed the yeast during this procedure. Therefore, do not consume any sugar or alcohol in any form. This includes all dairy, grains, and fruit. This is twenty days of a wonderful vegetable, nuts, seeds and sprouted legume diet; thus insuring a healthy life, free of Systemic Yeast Overgrowth.

Candida/Leaky Gut Syndrome Cleanse Schedule						
IS = Intestinal Sweep		LB = Lower Bowel		SD = Soothing Digestion		
	Date	7:00am	10:00am	1:00pm	4:00pm	7:00pm
Step 1 2 DAYS Intestinal Sweep IS=50 LB=12		5-IS/2-LB	5-IS	5-IS/2-LB	5-IS	5-IS/2-LB
	1					
	2					
		7:00am	10:00am	1:00pm	4:00pm	7:00pm
		5-SD/2-IS	5-SD	5-SD/2-IS	5-SD	5-SD/2-IS
Step 2 14 DAYS Soothing Digestion SD=350 13 DAYS Intestinal Sweep IS= 78	3					
	4					
	5					
	6					
	7					
	8					
	9					
	10					
	11					
	12					
	13					
	14					
	15					
	16					
		7:00am	10:00am	1:00pm	4:00pm	7:00pm
Step 3 2 DAYS Intestinal Sweep IS=50 LB=12		5-IS/2-LB	5-IS	5-IS/2-LB	5-IS	5-IS/2-LB
	17					
	18					
		7:00am	10:00am	1:00pm	4:00pm	7:00pm
	Select Probiotic of Choice	*Probiotics	*Probiotics	*Probiotics	*Probiotics	*Probiotics
Step 4 2 MOS Re-establish Flora: *Probiotics 3x label dosage or Large Amounts of: *Raw Sauerkraut *Kim Chi *Raw Apple Cider Vinegar *Rejuvelac *Miso	19					
Herbs required:	2 Bottles-Soothing Digestion		1 Bottle-Intestinal Sweep		1 Bottle-Lower Bowel	

Notes: You should have 3 bowel movements a day. This is most important during the first procedure so that the body is eliminating the yeast, etc... If necessary, the Lower Bowel formula can be taken the entire time. In some cases, a colonic might be necessary.

Figure 6

CANDIDA MENU PLAN

Monday
Breakfast: Oatmeal(using the thermos method) with almond milk(unsweetened) add tsp of cinnamon Sprinkle on some hulled hemp seeds.
Midmorning: juice with celery, parsley, and spinach
Lunch: salad with mixed greens, cucumber with garlic, lemon, olive and flax oil dressing. 1 carrot and 1celery stick. Hand full of walnuts.
Dinner: Tempeh or Tofu (organic or GMO free) stir fry with brown rice and tahini sauce, grilled/baked vegetables (zucchini, onion, garlic, and squash) green salad with a garlic, lemon and olive oil dressing.
Tuesday
Breakfast: Oatmeal(using the thermos method) with almond milk(unsweetened) add tsp of cinnamon
Midmorning: juice with cucumber, 1 carrot, parsley
Lunch: Green salad or bean salad (no sugar), avocado, green onion with garlic and oil, grilled vegetables
Dinner: Vegan Sushi rolls(use brown rice only) made with avocado, carrot and mushroom. Green salad made with Tahini dressing and sunflower seeds)
Wednesday
Breakfast: Oatmeal(using the thermos method) with almond milk(unsweetened) add tsp of cinnamon
Midmorning: juice with celery, parsley, and mixed greens
Lunch: Green salad with spinach, sunflower seeds, cucumber, with garlic, lemon, ginger and olive oil dressing.
Dinner: vegan pattie on 2 slices of Ezekiel bread or Vegetable Quinoa, Add slice of tomato, Mushrooms, onion with 2 carrot and celery sticks. Green salad with tahini dressing.
Thursday
Breakfast: Oatmeal(using the thermos method) with almond milk(unsweetened) add tsp of cinnamon.
Midmorning: juice with cucumber, parsley, and spinach
Lunch: Green salad with cabbage, green onion, 1/2 grated carrot, with ginger, oil, lemon, garlic, and dill for dressing, hand full of walnuts.

Dinner: grilled or steamed vegetables over brown rice. Sliced tomato 1 slice of Ezekiel bread. Hummus with radishes or celery.

Friday

Breakfast: Oatmeal(using the thermos method) with almond milk(unsweetened) add tsp of cinnamon.

Midmorning: juice with celery, parsley.

Lunch: salad with Romaine Lettuce, avocado, green onion with Garlic and oil dressing, black bean soup with grilled vegetables

Dinner: Vegan burger sandwich(see above on what to add) or Vegetable Quinoa with a green salad or Sushi rolls.

You can also snack on black bean soup, parsley soup, and vegetable broth in rotation. It is fine to mix and match.

The above menu plan is an example. Mondays do not have be Monday, Tuesdays do not have to be Tuesday. You can mix and swap individual meals. Also, the weekend, Saturday and Sunday, also use the same meals. The most important thing to take from this is if it (food) is on the menu plan, you can eat it. If it is not, than you cannot. You are attempting to starve the candida while the holistic medications eradicate it.

If you like you can add PLAIN(NOSUGAR) plant yogurt to any of the days. Maybe have a cup for breakfast instead of Oatmeal or add it with the oatmeal.

    **For your yogurt you can add a few walnuts or sunflower seeds.
    **Hummous can be used on the vegan burgers or use as a dressing.

DIETARY/NUTRITION:

Once the candida cleanse is done, the patient is then instructed to follow a strict but diverse vegan diet. This is duet o t several reasons. This allows for a significantly reduced mucous-less diet raising the pH of the patient and allowing less mucous for the bacteria to feed upon. It also drastically lowers the arachidonic acid levels. Lowering this EFA has been found to dramatically decrease the amount of systemic inflammation, thereby lowering the level of joint pain in the patient, a very common symptom of Lyme.

Part of the program entails nutrition education whereby we supply the patient with vegan menu plans, nutrition charts detailing foods high in protein, calcium, magnesium, potassium and other naturally occurring vitamins and minerals.

MEDICATION (STANDARD AMONGST ALL PATIENTS):
Holistic medication is second to nutrition in this program. As I tell the patients, holistic medications can work very well but they have ot have something, building blocks, to work with and that comes from nutrition. One of the first assessments for a proper Lyme program is to ascertain the patient's list of symptoms, which then enables the practitioner to define some of the collateral damage done by the disease. In most case, this presents as joint and muscle pain, nerve damage, heart issues if they have had the disease for a significantly long period of time, fatigue, and malnutrition.

We start all Lyme patients with a standard list of holistic medications (herbal and vitamin/minerals) along with bowel and liver cleansing herbs.

BOWEL CLEANSING AND SUPPORT:
Barberry bark (Berberis vulgaris), Cascara sagrada bark (Rhamnus purshiana), Cayenne (Capsicum minimum), Ginger (Zingiber officinale) Golden seal root (Hydrastis canadensis), Lobelia herb and/or seeds (Lobelia inflata), Red raspberry leaves (Rubus idaeus), Turkey rhubarb root (Rheum palmatum), Fennel (Foeniculum vulgari)

LIVER AND GALLBLADDER SUPPORT:

The herbs that compose the liver-gallbladder formula are: barberry, wild yam, cramp bark, fennel seed, ginger, catnip and peppermint.

BLOOD CLEANSING:
Red clover blossoms, chaparral, licorice root, poke root, peach bark, Oregon grape root, stillingia, prickly ash bark, burdock root, and buckthorn bark.

JOINT PAIN:

This usually involves two separate holistic medications:
For joint repair:
Hydrangea root Brigham herb yucca chaparral black walnut, lobelia burdock root, sarsaparilla wild lettuce Valerian wormwood cayenne black cohosh.
For pain and inflammation: Willow tincture.
FOR THE BACTERIAL: INFECTION:
As mentioned earlier in this paper, Cat's Claw is the main "natural antibiotic" used in the battle against the Lyme bacteria. Garlic is also extensively used.

MEDICATION (UNIQUE TO EACH PATIENT BASED ON THE DAMAGE DONE):

For heart damage: Ingredients: Hawthorn berry syrup is made with hawthorn berry juice concentrate using grape brandy and glycerin as aids and preservatives.

For Nerve damage: Ingredients: Black cohosh capsicum hops flowers lobelia skullcap Valerian wood betony mistletoe. I also use one that is used as ear drops: Ingredients: black cohosh blue cohosh blue Vervain skullcap lobelia.

SAUNA, EXERCISE FOR OXYGEN AND HEAT TREATMENTS:
One if the characteristics about the Lyme bacteria is it's intolerance for heat and oxygen. It is now an accepted protocol for Lyme patients to exercise each week, starting at about an a week and building up. This is meant to be strenuous aerobic exercises causing the patients body heat to increase as well as their oxygen load. Most patients report a small Herx response right after the session. For those not able to exercise effectively, a sauna has been found to work well.

Sauna therapy. The Lyme spirochete appears to be very heat sensitive. This is a fact we use to our advantage with near infrared light sauna therapy. It works beautifully with many cases of Lyme disease, and is inexpensive and completely non-toxic. I recommend at least two lamp sauna sessions daily, and they should be 45 to 60 minutes long at 120 degrees F.

FURTHER MEDICATION FOR PAIN:

A combination of Cramp bark and Valerian is used in tincture form as a very powerful and effective muscle relaxer and pain killer. Willow is a very good choice for minor pain and as an anti-inflammatory. CBD in the form of capsules, oils and salves works wonderfully as a quick and efficient pain killer. But again, the best pain killer is finding a cure for the disease.

STRESS MANAGEMENT:

Many different studies lend insight to the role of stress on patients with chronic illness. It is observed that stress also may affect the progression of infection and infectious disease. Research findings have continuously demonstrated a significant role that stress has in bacterial, viral and fungal infection, leading one to conclude that stress is a significant factor in susceptibility, severity, and progression of disease and illness. A growing body of evidence indicates that stress can make arthritis pain worst by increasing sensitivity to pain, reducing coping efforts, and possibly affecting the process of inflammation itself, these direct effects occur through neuroendocrine responses to stress. Stress plays a huge role in chronic illness. Stress is defined as the physical or mental response to demands from the environment, the events that led up to these demands, or the individual's perception of these demands.
If the need is great enough I will recommend talk therapy to give the patient an avenue in dealing with the serious internal issues. I will also discuss various coping mechanisms such as exercise, walking on the forest (also called Forest Bathing by the Japanese), finding hobbies they have not done in years, building a circle of close friends and support groups, both local and online.

LABS FOR MONITORING PROGRESS OF TREATMENT:

As mentioned earlier in this book, the two primary blood test I use for diagnosing and monitoring the progression of the treatment is the Western Blood Serum test and the CD57. Many doctors not trained in Lyme will often opt for the Western Blot Reflex test. This is a very significant mistake as it's success rate for detecting the Lyme bacteria is very poor. Lyme trained doctors will avoid this test and opt for the Serum version.

12.3 Case Histories

CASE HISTORY #1
Heather – Lyme Disease

One of the joys we get at the clinic is the opportunity to be one of the only Lyme-literate clinics in Northern California. It is a sad state to find how little is known about this disease and how poorly the CDC encourages information. It is terribly under reported due to the CDC requirements being absurdly high for what can be classified as Lyme disease.

Fortunately we have Dr. Christopher's knowledge and that of Dr. Burascano, the worlds leading authority on Lyme Disease. He is also very open to alternative medicine as an option for treatment. He has treated over 11,000 patients worldwide. Heather is a common example of a patient with Lyme Disease. Rarely does the patient receive treatment shortly after being bitten by the deer tick as this creature is quite small and most patients will not even realize they have been bitten. In only 20% of the cases does the classic "target" rash show up. In her case she was not diagnosed until about nine years after he initial infection. This results in what we classify as chronic or late term Lyme Disease with secondary infections. This usually results in chronic joint and muscle pain, fatigue, a suppressed immune system along with a variety of other symptoms.

She had been constantly misdiagnosed and was usually labeled with Chronic Fatigue Syndrome, a blanket diagnosis meaning they have no idea what is happening to the patient.

In her case we finally received a blood test back called the Western Blot Test. It showed the bacteria markers for the Lyme Disease organism. We began treatment immediately. One of the most important things to do for chronic Lyme Disease is to deal with the long term damage which is usually with the nerves. We also have to be careful treating the disorder too aggressively as a large die-off of the bacteria can actually harm the patient. We started with the three day cleanse using carrot juice and afterwards she adopted the mucousless diet. The cleansing formulas Lower Bowel and Liver and Gallbladder along with the Kidney formula were also utilized.

To aid in the nerve and joint damage we also added the formulas MindTrac, Relax-Eze, St. John's Wort, Complete Tissue and Bone and the Joint formula. To aid in the compromised immune system we added the Adrenal Formula with Immucalm. Within the first month on the program she noticed an increased energy and a lessening of the joint and muscle pain. Her physician in her area has asked for us to consult with him so he can better treat his other patients with this issue. While this program usually takes about a year to complete she continues to improve to this day.

CASE HISTORY #2:
Lara

The patient is a 33 year female who originally came to the clinic presenting a diagnosis of multiple sclerosis. I accepted the previous doctor's assessment and began treating her for this condition. Over the period of a year she saw significant improvement gaining the ability to move out on her own for the first and to hold down a job. Within three weeks of treatment she was no longer using her cane. Since she was doing so well we discontinued the monthly visits and asked her to watch her diet, which was vegan, and to let us know how she was doing. About a year later we saw her again and her old symptoms were returning. I asked if she would be willing to take a series of Lyme blood test and she agreed. The results came back positive. She had been misdiagnosed all along.

We began the outlined Lyme protocol and within weeks she was noticing significant improvement and her CD57 blood test continues to rise. By 07/18/2018 the CD57 increased to 105 from a previous value of 72 back in April.

CASE HISTORY #3:
Marci

This patient was a 45 year old woman presenting advanced chronic Lyme disease. Symptoms were burning skin, extensive joint and muscle pain, gut issues, weak muscles and systemic candida.

The first protocol involved our 18 day candida cleanse which at the end the patient already noted some improvement in the joint pain. She remained vegan at this point and began the protocol of holistic medication mentioned in this paper along with weekly exercise and saunas. Her energy continued to improve as well a her anxiety and depression disappeared.

She experienced extensive Herxx reactions when I started her later n the Cat's Claw but in time this has significantly disappeared as I increased the dosages. Her latest Western blot showed only one marker remaining. Her last CD57 had risen to a 105 which indicated her immune was starting to fight back successfully.

CASE HISTORY #4:
Donna

This patient was a 53 year old woman who originally presented a very serious case of vaginitis. I ran an STD test and it came back as HSV type 1. She also presented a suppressed immune system, allergies, systemic candida, and painful joints.

She went through the 18 day candida protocol and noticed a slight improvement in her energy and joints. I then proceeded to treat the HSV 1 rash vaginally with immune supporting herbs and St. John's Wort, both internally and topically.

The rash improved but it was a very slow process.
She mentioned an issue with a tick bit in her past so I arraigned for a complete Lyme blood test. The Western Blot Serum showed two bands and the CD57 was a 21, an extremely low value and highly indicative of chronic Lyme.

We started the full Lyme program and in six months her CD57 climbed to a 67, indicating her immune system was beginning to rally. Her vaginitis completely vanished along with a significant improvement in her energy and no longer had any joint pain.

CHAPTER 13

Complimentary results compared with conventional

Conventional: Post-Treatment Lyme Disease Syndrome (PTLDS) represents a subset of patients who remain significantly ill following standard antibiotic therapy for Lyme disease. PTLDS is characterized by a constellation of symptoms that includes severe fatigue, musculoskeletal pain, sleep disturbance, depression, and cognitive problems such as difficulty with short-term memory, speed of thinking, or multi-tasking. In the absence of a direct diagnostic biomarker, PTLDS has been difficult to diagnose by physicians, and its existence has been controversial. However, our clinical research shows that meticulous patient evaluation when used alongside appropriate diagnostic testing can reliably identify patients with typical symptom patterns of PTLDS. Our research also indicates that PTLDS symptoms can significantly impair daily functioning and quality of life. Increased severity of initial illness, the presence of neurologic symptoms, and initial misdiagnosis increase the risk of Post-Treatment Lyme Disease Syndrome. PTLDS is especially common in people that have had neurologic involvement. The rates of Post-Treatment Lyme Disease Syndrome after neurologic involvement may be as high as 20% or even higher. Without neurologic symptoms, the rates of Post-Treatment Lyme Disease Syndrome tend to be in the 10% to 20% range.

Complementary: Holistic treatment should entail well-selected remedies, including clinical chosen for the patient, intercurrent miasmatic remedies and acute remedies for side effects and die-off symptoms. These remedies should be changed according to the patient's responses. Then once 75% of the symptoms are taken care of and the patients can manage the acute flair ups (which should lessen in frequency after time as their health is restored) the Lyme disease is eradicated and their health is restored. At that point constitutional remedies should be prescribed at least once a year to maintain the patient's health.

In each of my patients who followed the program as prescribed, we saw 100% success with eradication of the symptoms as well as any sign clinically of the bacteria's presence.

References – Misdiagnosis of Lyme disease

1. Goldenberg DL. Fibromyalgia, chronic fatigue syndrome, and myofascial pain syndrome. Curr Opin Rheumatol, 6(2), 223-233 (1994).

2. Clauw DJ, Chrousos GP. Chronic pain and fatigue syndromes: overlapping clinical and neuroendocrine features and potential pathogenic mechanisms. Neuroimmunomodulation, 4(3), 134-153 (1997).

3. Naesens R, Vermeiren S, Van Schaeren J, Jeurissen A. False positive Lyme serology due to syphilis: report of 6 cases and review of the literature. Acta Clin Belg, 66(1), 58-59 (2011).

4. Cimmino MA, Salvarani C. Polymyalgia rheumatica and giant cell arteritis. Baillieres Clin Rheumatol, 9(3), 515-527 (1995).

5. Paparone PW. Polymyalgia rheumatica or Lyme disease? How to avoid misdiagnosis in older patients. Postgrad Med, 97(1), 161-164, 167-170 (1995).

6. Schwartzberg M, Weber CA, Musico J. Lyme borreliosis presenting as a polymyalgia rheumatica-like syndrome. Br J Rheumatol, 34(4), 392-393 (1995).

7. Daoud KF, Barkhuizen A. Rheumatic mimics and selected triggers of fibromyalgia. Curr Pain Headache Rep, 6(4), 284-288 (2002).

8. Steere AC, Malawista SE, Snydman DR et al. Lyme arthritis: an epidemic of oligoarticular arthritis in children and adults in three connecticut communities. Arthritis Rheum, 20(1), 7-17 (1977).

9. Feder HM, Jr., Whitaker DL. Misdiagnosis of erythema migrans. Am J Med, 99(4), 412-419 (1995).

10. Nowakowski J, McKenna D, Nadelman RB et al. Failure of treatment with cephalexin for Lyme disease. Arch Fam Med, 9(6), 563-567 (2000).

11. Plotkin SA. Correcting a public health fiasco: The need for a new vaccine against Lyme disease. Clinical infectious diseases : an official publication of the Infectious Diseases Society of America, 52 Suppl 3, s271-275 (2011).

12.Brinar VV, Habek M. Rare infections mimicking MS. Clin Neurol Neurosurg, (2010).

13.Calabresi PA. Diagnosis and management of multiple sclerosis. Am Fam Physician, 70(10), 1935-1944 (2004).

14.Trojano M, Paolicelli D. The differential diagnosis of multiple sclerosis: classification and clinical features of relapsing and progressive neurological syndromes. Neurol Sci, 22 Suppl 2, S98-102 (2001).

15.Fallon BA, Keilp JG, Corbera KM et al. A randomized, placebo-controlled trial of repeated IV antibiotic therapy for Lyme encephalopathy. Neurology, 70(13), 992-1003 (2008).

16.Paparone PW. Polymyalgia rheumatica or Lyme disease? How to avoid misdiagnosis in older patients. Postgrad Med, 97(1), 161-164, 167-170 (1995).

17.Schwartzberg M, Weber CA, Musico J. Lyme borreliosis presenting as a polymyalgia rheumatica-like syndrome. Br J Rheumatol, 34(4), 392-393 (1995).

18. Jennings F, Lambert E, Fredericson M. Rheumatic diseases presenting as sports-related injuries. Sports Med, 38(11), 917-930 (2008).

19. Cameron DJ. Consequences of treatment delay in Lyme disease. J Eval Clin Pract, 13(3), 470-472 (2007).

Hu LT. Lyme Disease. Ann Intern Med. 2016 Nov 1;165(9):677.

- Kowalski TJ, Tata S, Berth W, Mathiason MA, Agger WA Antibiotic treatment duration and long-term outcomes of patients with early Lyme disease from a Lyme disease-hyperendemic area. Clin Infect Dis. 2010;50(4):512-520.

- Sanchez E, Vannier E, Wormser GP, Hu LT. Diagnosis, treatment, and prevention of Lyme disease, human granulocytic anaplasmosis, and babesiosis: A review. JAMA. 2016 Apr 26;315(16):1767-77.

- Stupica D, Lusa L, Ruzić-Sabljić E, Cerar T, Strle F. Treatment of erythema migrans with doxycycline for 10 days versus 15 days. Clin Infect Dis. 2012;55(3):343-350.

PART FOUR – CASE HISTORIES FROM A SUCCESSFUL NATUROPATHIC CLINIC

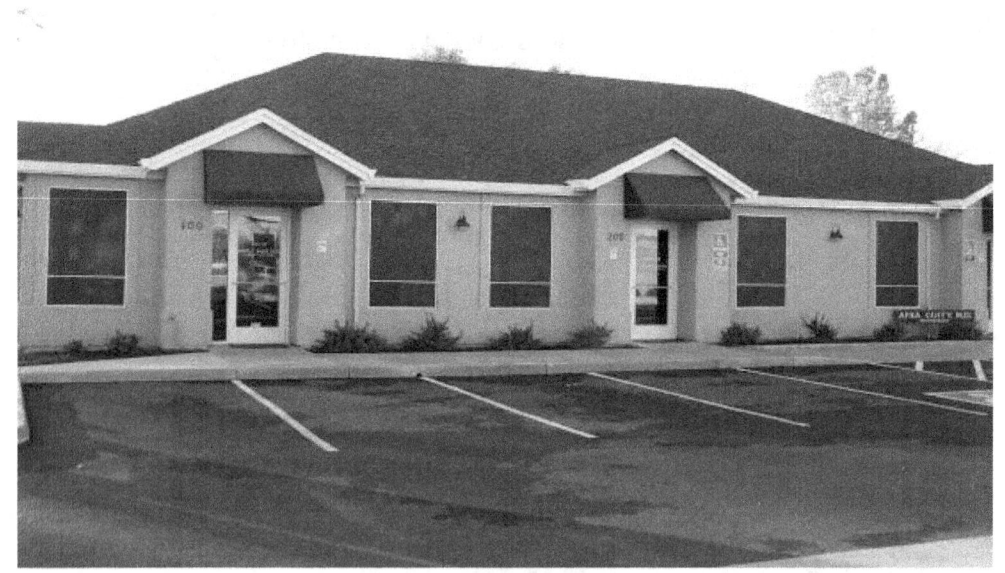

Introduction

The purpose of this book is to offer hope for an alternative treatment for chronic disease. The information contained describes in a small detail some of the work and case histories I have personally witnessed in my 20+ years of practice as an alternative healthcare provider. You will find a wide variety of cases ranging from simple cuts and wounds to serious auto-immune disorders such as Multiple Sclerosis and type 1 diabetes along with successful treatments for cancer.

You will notice as a common theme throughout each of these cases an overriding need for cleansing and dietary and lifestyle changes. This displays a single important point for ridding our bodies of disorder, cleansing it and making the appropriate changes so we do not end up back in the old condition. It is interesting to note that a survey was done by the AMA of all physicians who treat cancer. It was a one questions survey.

Each physician who had cancer patients in remission was to ask their patients if they had changed their lifestyles or diet having "survived" cancer. Even the AMA was stunned at the results. Over 90% percent came back and stated that they had not changed their lives in any manner. Hence, the reason cancer has a return rate of about five years and usually with a vengeance. This is actually not unexpected when you realize that only 6% percent of all U.S. physicians have had even a single semester credit of nutritional education out of eight years of higher education. That leaves us with 94% of all U.S. physicians with no education in nutrition, even though congress mandated that they receive said education. Today only half of all medical universities require this course.

It is in part because of this lack of knowledge on the doctor's behalf that illness continues to spread in the World's wealthiest nations. According to Clinic Compare out of Britain, they analyzed 179 countries based on information from the World Health Organization. America is the only non-European country to make the top 10 on the list, having the ninth highest rate of obesity in the world — 35% of the adult population is classified as dangerously overweight. It is considered the sickest nation in the developed World. As well as from other studies the results surprised even the researchers. To their alarm, they said, they found a "strikingly consistent and pervasive" pattern of poorer health at all stages of life, from infancy to childhood to adolescence to young adulthood to middle and old age. Compared to people in other developed nations, Americans die far more often from injuries and homicides. We suffer more deaths from alcohol and other drugs, and endure some of the worst rates of heart disease, lung disease, obesity, and diabetes.

Among the most striking of the findings are that, among the countries studied, the U.S. has:

- The highest rate of death by violence, by a stunning margin

- The highest rate of death by car accident, also dramatically so

- The highest chance that a child will die before age 5

- The second-highest rate of death by coronary heart disease

- The second-highest rate of death by lung disease

- The highest teen pregnancy rate

- The highest rate of women dying due to complications of pregnancy and childbirth

According to Pure Wellness out of the U.K., the United States has one of the worst diets in the World. As stated on their website:
"…where every portion of food or drink can be'super-sized'. This is the world of plenty! But where did it all go wrong for this nation? According to the documentary, it all started back in 1971 where President Nixon was hopeful for a re-election. Many Americans at the time were very unhappy about the high cost of food. So to get the price down, Nixon encouraged farmers to mass produce crops……and one in particular—**corn!** This process created a new product called **high fructose corn syrup (HFCS)**—A cheap sugar sweetener that can be

found in thousands of food products today. However, it didn't just stay in America. This processed product spread like wild fire to other countries with similar dieting problems such as… ".

Stress levels are also on the rise. A recent report shows America to be among the most stressed out nations on Earth. People are becoming more and more disconnected from the natural world and spending their lives in an environment devoid of tress, grass and open, quiet spaces.

So, what can be done about it? We need to take back control of our own lives and start caring for ourselves. As some wise folks have said in the past "Start eating like an adult". Start making healthy choices for yourself and that can start with a vegan diet. Organizations such as the World Health Organization, The U.N., Kaiser Permanente, the American College Of Lifestyle Medicine, The Physicians Committee for Responsible Medicine, Academy of Nutrition and Dietetics, The Mayo Clinic and many, many more recommend a plant-based diet.

We can also start looking for more natural alternatives for treating our selves and out families. While it is slowly increasing in the U.S., countries such as in Europe have been using herbal medications for thousands of years. To this day, you can go to a pharmacy in England and half of it will be pharmaceuticals and the other half stocked in natural medications. Physicians in Germany will prescribe St. John's Wort 90% of time over Prozac while the opposite is true in the States. Germany was so interested in proving the efficacy of herbal medications that their equivalent to the U.S. FDA funded a massive research project called the German Commission E. This study proved the efficacy of 380 different herbal substances.

Within these pages you will find holistic medicine's tried and true protocols used successfully for each and every type of condition. Whether I have a patient come in with a cold or cancer I basically treat them the same. Our clinic has gown throughout the years to being the most successful holistic clinic in Northern California because we follow Dr. Christopher's recommendations. Over the years I have seen thousands of patients and cannot take the time to list all of the wonderful people I have met. I will try and cover some of the more memorable here in this book. The names have been changed to protect their medical privacy.

CHAPTER 14

ACCIDENTS

14.1 Peggy Knives

You will notice several case histories detailing a particular patient by the name of Peggy. I must say that she is both my wife and my Herbal Poster Child. She has probably given me more practice than any patient in my 16 year history. This particular case history details a couple of very serious wounds.

Case History #1 Knife wound:

One afternoon my wife was at the house while I was with patients at the clinic. She had finished washing the dishes and they had been drying in the dish drain, yes, some folks still do that.

When the time came to put the silverware away she reached and grabbed several at the same time. Within the group was a knife pointing downward. While she was moving to the drawer the knife slipped out and embedded itself into her exposed foot.

She looked down and saw the knife sticking straight up with a little blood seeping from the point of impact. She knew as soon as she removed the knife the blood would flow. Fortunately, she kept the cayenne tincture we had made nearby. She removed the knife and the blood began to spurt from the wound.

She immediately placed about a dropper full of the tincture on her tongue and noticed within 30 seconds that the bleeding came to a stop. While the cayenne may be very hot it causes no tissue damage and it can be a very successful treatment for bleeding.

Case History #2 Vegetable slicer:

About a week prior to the previous event Peggy was slicing up a zucchini for my meal. Again, I was not at home but her having graduated from the Family Herbalist course prepared her for emergencies such as this one.

While slicing the vegetable she grew impatient. With only a slice or two remaining to be done she removed the blade guard to speed up the process. The very next slice removed a significant portion of her thumb at the tip. This produced a heart beat spurting of blood from the wound.

She immediately ran and retrieved the cayenne from our medicine shelves. She orally took about a dropper full and also poured some of the cayenne tincture on the counter and rubbed the wound in it. Needless to say, the pain was significant, but again, no tissue damage.

As she watched, the blood flow rapidly diminished and within about 60 seconds it had slowed to a gentle ooze.

14.2 Peggy - Burns

Again we return to my favorite patient, my wife Peggy. This event occurred due to an extremely overheated wax women use for their bikini area.

As usual, I was not at home when this occurred but due to her education with the School of Natural Healing she knew what to do.

She was microwaving wax and left it in too long. She had also been using the same plastic container for years and it had degraded. When she pulled the wax out of the oven the bottom collapsed and the molten wax poured onto her leg and foot.

The resulting effect was a second degree burn, just shy of third degree. She knew to immediately get the B, F and C salve out of the refrigerator and tried to apply it to the burn but unfortunately the wax had seared to the flesh and could not be removed.

She called me and I rushed back to the house. I found her on the floor in pain. I helped her into the living room where I then applied a very generous amount of the salve straight onto the top and surrounding area of the wax. Within minutes the salve began to seep under the wax and the pain diminished.

Within about 40 minutes enough of the salve had worked it's way under the wax and we were able to simply lift it off of her foot. Underneath was a very serious deep burn. We applied more salve and over the next two weeks she would reapply it and bandage.

In the end, the burn completely healed with no lasting scarring. Needless to say, that was the end of waxing.

14.3 Bob - Gangrene

This was most likely the worst case of gangrene with extensive tissue necrosis I have ever had to treat. I had treated this patient in the past for various simple issues and had not seen him in about eight months. He called me on a Sunday requesting I make a house call as soon as possible. He stated he had damaged his foot back in November of the previous year and it was now early January.

I arrived at his house to find a foot in the early stages of gangrene. The flesh had begun to turn red, phasing towards brown. He had an elevated temperature and a rapid heart beat. The foot had become greatly swollen with an extensive flow of pus and lymph from the small wound on the bottom pad. The smell in the house was almost unbearable.

He stated the original wound was from a simple tack stepped on in the back yard that Fall. Something told me to check his blood sugar. I had never treated him for diabetes but I went ahead and checked. He had a blood glucose level of 300. Here we had a very serious situation of uncontrolled diabetes. He was in great danger of losing his foot as well as going into septic shock.

He stated he would not go to the hospital so we began treatment on the spot. I cleaned the wound and began applying herbal antiseptics. The formula used we call Herbadyne, the herbal sister to Betadine. It contains Myrrh, Goldenseal and Cayenne. It does sting just like Iodine. After this we dressed the initial wound in B, F and C salve.

For the systemic infection, we put him on Garlic at five capsules every hour. We also included the formula **Infection** from Dr. Christopher at the same dosage. He was also given Echinacea/Goldenseal at 4 capsules 4 times a day.

He was also instructed to eat as much raw garlic each day as he could stand, usually in the form of Dr. Christopher's Flu Stew. The Blood Stream formula was also administered each day at 4 droppers 5 times a day to cleanse the infection from his blood.

To aid in rebuilding the massive tissue loss, both skin and muscle, he was instructed to take B, F and C at 5 capsules 5 times a day.

To combat the gangrene, he was to soak his foot in an Epsom bath with a decoction of Marshmallow and Lobelia two to three times a day, soaking for a half hour or more. B, F and C fomentations were also used at night. During the day, the same salve was kept on the bottom of the foot.

After about a month the wound on the bottom of the foot began to seal but the infection was far from over. With nowhere for the infection to go the body found a way. Skin eruptions began to occur on the top of the foot. The patient and his wife called them little volcanoes. They could watch the eruption swell over the course of a day and then finally they would burst and the infection would literally flow out. It was the **Blood Steam** formula which aided in finding an avenue for the infection to leave the body.

Around the second month we began to apply a plantain poultice to the top of the foot where the eruptions where occurring. He was to continue with the previous treatment except the new poultice was to be kept on all night. This finally turned the tide and the infection began to diminish.

All told, it took about three months for the greater part of the healing to occur. The patient and his wife had stated to me, due to past experience with other family members, that if we had not followed the type of treatment protocol, a hospital would have removed several toes, if not the entire foot. Below are a serious of pictures demonstrating the healing.

His recovery has been a blessing. Because of the extensive use of the B, F and C he noticed that his old back injury was healed and can now even lift weights again. His diabetes also shows signs of healing as he is now completely off his diabetic medication.

Be warned, they are graphic.

The first week of treatment
Initial wound

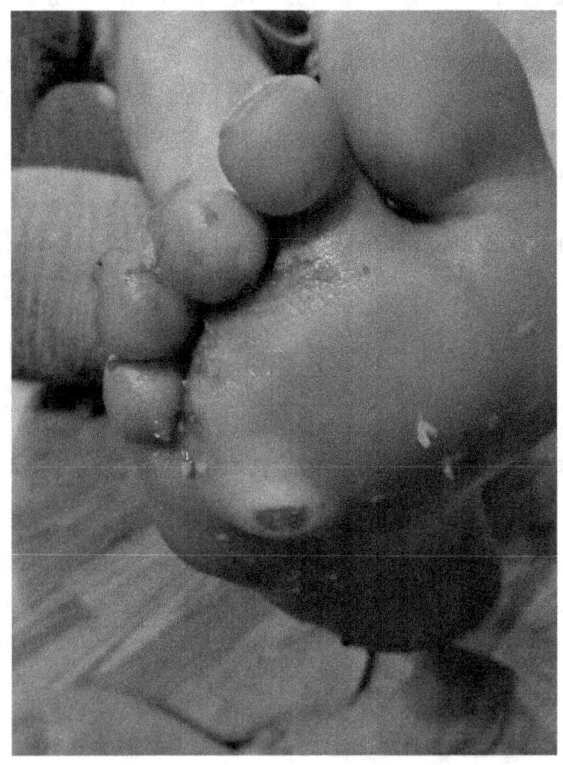

The First Month

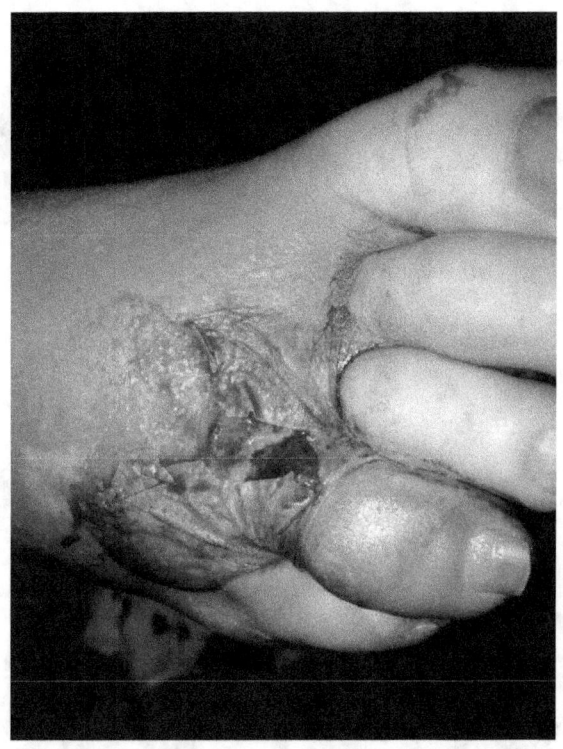

A closer look

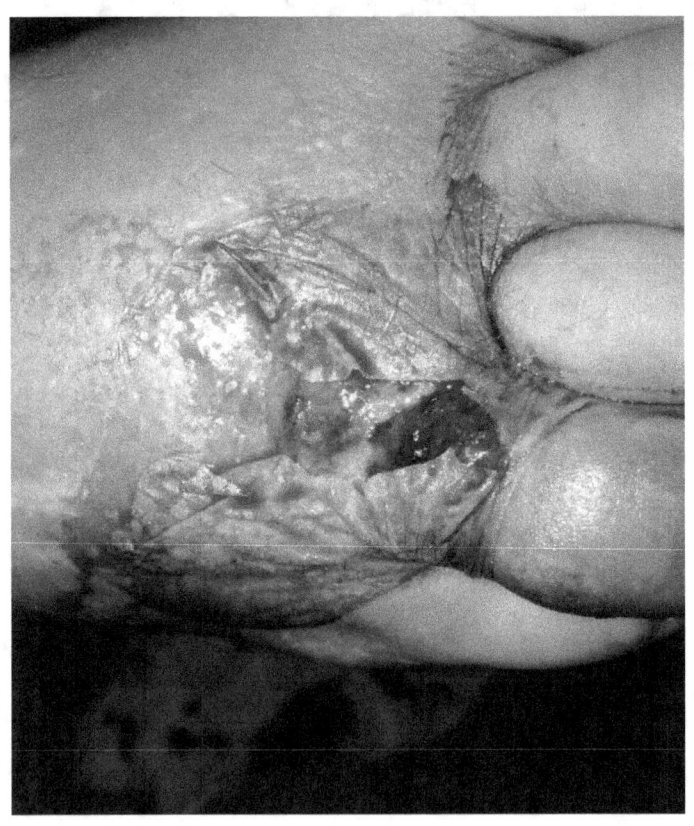

Two months into treatment

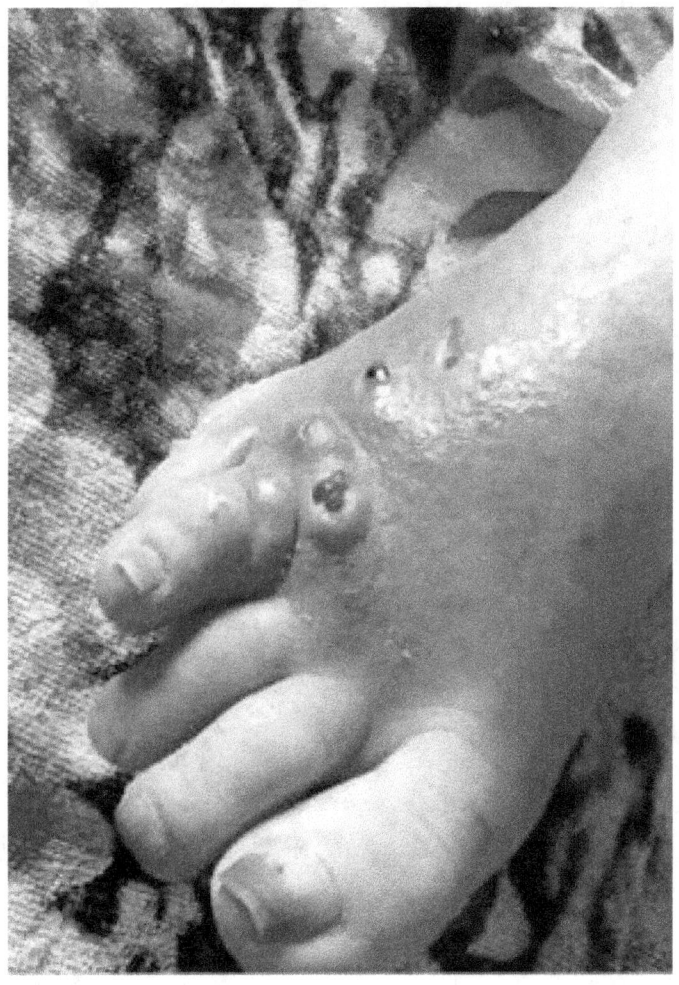

First Week of May

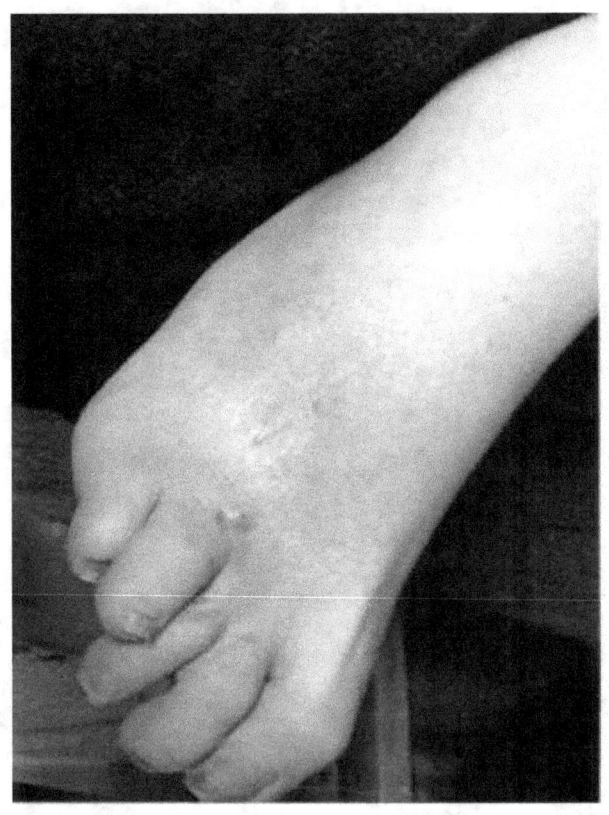

CHAPTER 15

Children

15.1 Jill – Pregnancy

This has to stand out as one of the most wonderful and moving cases I have had in reference to pregnancy. Jill is a current patient with the clinic and originally came to us to treat her children for such minor issues as colds and bronchitis. Then one day she announced she was pregnant and wanted us to assist in the pregnancy to insure a healthy baby and delivery. She currently uses a midwife and plans for a home water delivery.

One morning she called the clinic during her 11th week and stated she was spotting. We asked her to immediately come in. Upon arrival we had a very distraught mommy to be and we did a basic exam over the abdomen and listened for the baby. At this point we did not see anything wrong so we ran an ultrasound to check on the child. The joy in her face when we showed her a bouncy baby with a strong heartbeat made the rest of my week a happy one.

We still were not sure what was causing the bleeding so we dispensed to her Dr. Christopher's Anti-Miscarriage formula consisting of False Unicorn and Lobelia. Within twenty four hours she reported that the bleeding had stopped. What she reported next was nothing short of a miracle.

Within the first day or two of using the formula she felt something passing through her cervix. A small bean sized, gel encased sack was expelled which she promptly took to her midwife. The midwife informed her it was an eight week old fetus that had passed and that Jill had been carrying it alongside the healthy fetus.

The anti-miscarriage formula had caused her to expel the fetus which had passed several weeks earlier, while saving the healthy fetus. Currently, she is having a very healthy pregnancy and is still taking the anti-miscarriage formula.

17 Mar 2015

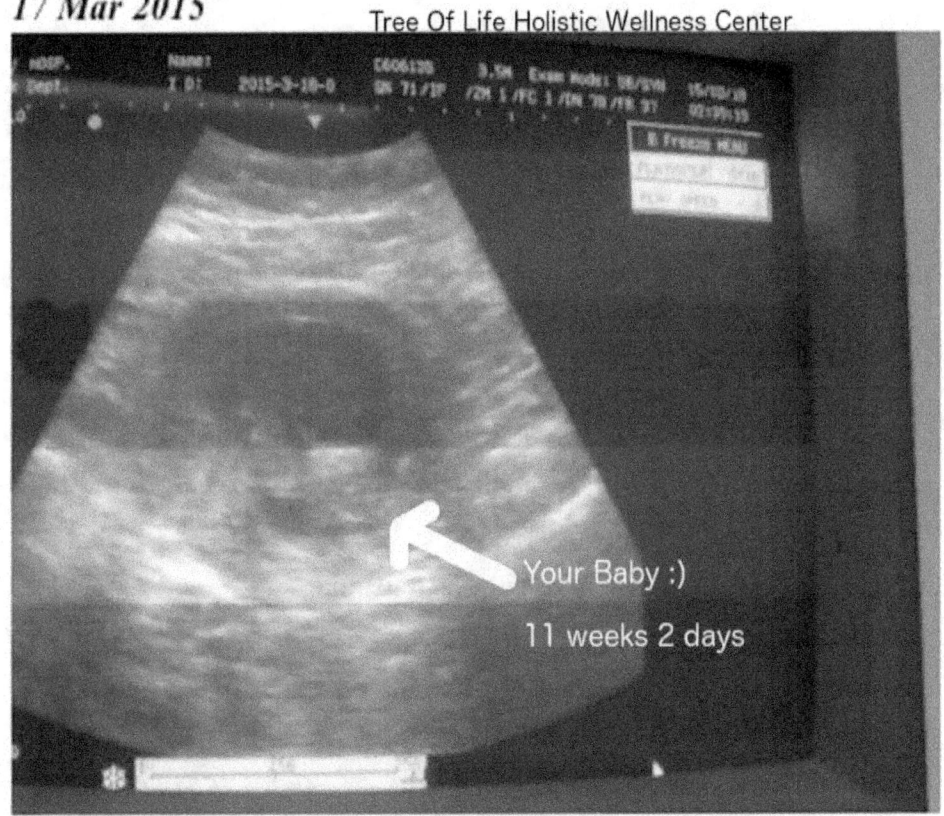

15.2 Jane – Pregnancy

Jane is one of those cases that you will remember for the rest of your life as it contains the gift of new life. She came to us shortly after I had started my career as a Master Herbalist. She had been told she could never have a child as she could not safely carry to term.

We told her there is no such thing as an incurable disease and that nothing was written in stone. She started the incurables program with a mucousless, vegan diet and began using the Formulas **Lower Bowel**, and **Liver and Gallbladder** while drinking plenty of Red Raspberry tea.

We also put her on the formulas Female Reproductive and Hormonal Changese with wheatgerm oil. Prior to starting the herbal therapy she also did the three day cleanse using carrot juice. We find carrot juice one of the best liver cleansers in nature.

After about eight months on this program we recommended that if she chose to she could try again to become pregnant. She did in fact become pregnant quick quickly and nine months later gave birth to a beautiful little boy.

He is now about 14 years old and a gift to us all.

15.3 Mark – Impotent

This patient was actually a nephew in law and came to us with an issue of impotency. I knew him as a small child and he was one of those constantly picked on by his other cousins. When full grown he was quite tall and had decided he was no longer going to be abused. It was at that time he started taking steroids, synthetic testosterone. In the end he became a very large and muscular man. The ladies loved him.

Eventually he met the love of his life and they married. After about a year of marriage his wife asked him to stop taking the steroids as she knew they were very dangerous and put him at risk for such diseases as prostate and testicular cancer among a wide variety of other issues. He did as she asked.

This resulted in a complete lack of sex drive nor the ability to perform sexually. As we were taught at the School of Natural Healing, if you give the body something it should be making on it's own, it will stop making it. This resulted in the atrophying of the testicles and their shrinking.

We had him do a three day cleanse with carrot juice and stated the basic program using **Lower Bowel**, **Liver and Gallbladder**, **Blood Stream** and the glandular formula continuing Mullein and Lobelia.

Due to the severity of his case he was also told to use the Mullein and Lobelia as a fomentation directly on his testicles each night for six nights a week for many months. This was quite embarrassing for him as it required the use of a cloth diaper held in place while he watched TV each night.

I asked them to not try and have a child for at least one year. The wife also followed the basic program and ate better during this time.

In time he did heal and they were able to conceive and have a little baby girl.

15.4 "Cub" - Severe bronchitis

"Cub" was a six month old little boy who came into the clinic with sever bronchitis. This past Winter we saw so much of this we named it the "crud". It would always start as a simple cold and then progress into the chest.

We took his vitals and he did have a small fever and quite a bit of discharge from the sinuses. Since he was still breast-feeding we asked the mother to take garlic at a dosage of 4 capsules five times a day. For "Cub" we had her administer to him a dropper of Dr. Christopher's formula **Lung and Bronchial** along with the **Super Immune Garlic** extract. Children seem to do quite well with the flavor of both of these formulas.

We also instructed the mother how to do the onion poultice with olive oil on his little chest, to be done each day. The formula Sen Sei was also applied each day to aid in his breathing.

Within about two days he was showing remarkable recovery and in a week the issues were over.

UPDATE:

A few months later he came into the clinic with a serious issue of constipation. He had not had a bowel movement in four days. We asked the mother to give "Cub" the children's version of the liquid **Lower Bowel** and asked her to use it at a dosage of half a dropper twice a day. I told her to expect results within twenty-four hours.

She reported that after an hour of the first administering, done at the clinic, he had a very successful bowel movement and was much more regular from that point on.

15.5 John - Appendicitis

"John" was a nine year old boy with acute appendicitis. His parents had originally taken him to the hospital with sever pain in the lower right quadrant of his abdomen. He was diagnosed with acute appendicitis and was advised to have immediate surgery. The family had a serious financial issue and also did not believe in removing his appendix.

They called me late at night and requested our help as an emergency situation. They had pulled him out of the hospital and met me at the clinic.

We opened the clinic for them and made sure they understood the seriousness of the situation and asked if they were sure this is the path they wanted to take. They again requested our assistance so we began to treat him.

W immediately began to administer the formulas **Lower Bowel** and **Liver and Gallbladder**. We also asked the parents to administer catnip and fennel enemas which brought immediate relief from the pain.

For the rest of the night we had them use castor oil packs over the appendix area using the twelve minutes hot and four minutes cold routine. This also aided in relieving any pain the child was experiencing.

By the end of the night the pain was completely gone and the issue had passed. The parents later had him checked out and no sign of the appendicitis could be found. Yet another appendix saved from the surgeons knife.

15.6 Multiple Autism cases

We have had multiple cases of autism brought into our clinic over the past several years. I have little doubt that vaccines are the leading contributing factors behind these issues. No child that came into our clinic who has never received vaccines have we ever seen this issue present.

At our clinic we are able to run a urinalysis test for neurotransmitters. We can test for six different transmitters and this gives us a very clear understanding of what is happening within the brain. The test results for all autistic children are almost identical. They almost invariably show a significant imbalance in the chemicals of the brain, leading to OCD, attention disorders and a lack of social skills.

Our standard protocol utilizes a mucous-less diet, cleansing routines using the formulas **Lower Bowel** and **Liver and Gallbladder** . With this we add the following formulas **MindTrac** (or **Kid-e-Trac**), **Relax-Eze** and **St. John's Wort.**

Invariably, within a two month period of the children following the program we receive reports of the children's moods stabilizing, their attention spans increasing and the ability to sleep better at night. One particular mother reported to us that she felt she had her son back. We will go into this issue in greater detail when we discuss Nathan who had both psoriasis and autism.

15.7 Lisa – Morbid obesity and Pregnancy

This was a very rewarding case which stands as proof that even those patients with a high risk pregnancy can have a healthy and vibrant child. Our patient was a 24 year old female who was morbidly obese at 300+ pounds. She originally came to us with Polycsytic Ovarian Syndrome and was unable to conceive. We put her on the standard holistic program for female reproductive issues utilizing such herbal medications as Blessed Thistle, Red Raspberry tea, Black and Blue Cohosh, as well as colon and liver cleansing routines and a vegan diet.

She had issues with loosing weight due to a high stress life and turning to food for comfort. But, over time she did lose some of the weight and eventually did conceive. At this point no other doctor would work with her as she was considered such a high risk case. Morbid obesity during pregnancy can commonly lead to gestational diabetes causing the baby to become too large, placenta previa, high blood pressure and miscarriage, to name just a few.

We continued to treat her and to support the pregnancy. She stayed on at least a quart a day of Red Raspberry tea. I know that a simple search of the web gives grave warnings of drinking Red Raspberry tea during pregnancy but it is not true. All of our pregnant patients are put on this tea and have seen amazing results with a healthy pregnancy and babies.

We also put her on an anti-miscarriage formula utilizing False Unicorn and Lobelia. In an earlier case in this book I discuss the wonderful benefits of this formula and have never seen it fail in preventing miscarriage.

We monitored her throughout her pregnancy with blood work and ultrasounds each month. She remained on the vegan diet and after nine months delivered a beautiful baby girl and throughout her pregnancy did not have a single complication, as would have been predicted by most obstetricians.

15.8 Johnny – Almost fatal anemia – age 21 months

Sometimes a case will come to us that moves our hearts and stays with us long after the patient has been treated. This is a case of a very little boy who came very close to death with little advanced notice to his parents.

I received a call on our emergency line a Friday when the clinic was closed. It was from a very distraught mother calling from UC Davis fighting not to lose custody of her child to the hospital. Earlier that morning the child walking tough the house when he suddenly collapsed and was unable to move one side of his body. The parents immediately rushed him to the local hospital where they examined him and ran a blood test. The blood test revealed a hemoglobin level of a 4, a very dangerous level when a normal level for him would be more in the 12 range. The hospital evaced him down to US Davis oncology.

After receiving him, the hospital determined he needed an immediate blood transfusion. His parents are Jehovah's Witnesses and transfusion are against their faith so they declined. At this point the hospital notified them that if they refused they would remove the child from their custody and perform what procedures they felt necessary. The mother, whose mother and father were both patients of ours, called and asked for us to intervene to stop their child from being taken away from them.

I spoke with the hospital and told them I would take over the care of the child with the agreement that we would send weekly blood test results to them. Amazingly, they agreed. I spoke again with the mother and gave him some basic advice for the weekend and to bring him into the clinic on Monday. Since I was not sure what was the cause of his condition I asked for them to at least get him started on organic black strap molasses, a food extremely high in calcium and iron. We also had his blood test results sent to me immediately so I could review the case.

One of the most common mistakes many doctors make with anemia is the diagnosis that the patient is low on iron. This is actually usually not the case but simply one of a lack of assimilating the iron already present in the blood. What the blood test results revealed was a surprise to me. The child was actually in iron overload and the lab showed he was already experiencing kidney and liver damage. High iron in the blood can cause both liver and kidney damage. Originally, the hospitals thought it was a viral infection, which can cause these types of symptoms in little ones. A more detailed intake done at our clinic revealed that the mother had given him too may iron supplements, resulting in iron overload. If the hospital had given him the transfusion it most likely would have killed him, since he already had too much iron in his system resulting in kidney and liver damage.

We kept him on the black strap molasses and also started him on a dietary routine high in the minerals that better enable to the body to assimilate iron. We also also put him him on a natural, herbal iron formula. Again, this was not necessarily high in iron but in the minerals and vitamins required to assimilate what was already in his little body.

Each week we checked his hemoglobin levels and faxed them to UC Davis. Each week they continued to rise and within four weeks he was at normal levels. Almost immediately, his skin color improved as well as his energy level and he was quickly back to a very energetic 21 month old little boy.

CHAPTER 16

Lung Issues

16.1 William – COPD

William was an 89 year old patient with severe COPD and was dependent on an oxygen bottle to survive the night. He also required a rescue inhaler and various other asthma type medications.

He stated he was ready to get away from these medications as he knew they were very damaging to his liver. As always, we never have a patient get off of their medicaments as this could be very dangerous. We let their previous primary lower their dosage as they notice they no longer need them as much. Eventually they are usually able to get completely off of them.

He started the mucous-less diet after a very successful three day cleanse with carrot juice. He followed the cleansing program using **Lower Bowel**, **Liver and Gallbladder** with **Kidney** and **Blood Stream** added later. We also added the Lung and Bronchial formula along with a tincture made from Mullein and Lobelia to act as a bronchial dilator and anti-spasmodic.

We also used the formula **Complete Tissue and Bone** to aid in healing the lung tissue. After about two months he was off the oxygen bottle and by month three all of his medications were discontinued.

To this day he has not required any of our formulas or the previous medications. An interesting note, it took him about five months to get the oxygen company to come and pick up the bottles as the company did not want to lose the insurance payments.

16.2 Paul – Tuberculosis

Paul is an immigrant patient from Mexico who came into the United States as a nine year old child. At that time a TB test showed he was a carrier and was not active with the disease. This had a multitude of ramifications for him in such areas as getting employment and citizenship. He brought in a blood test which proved he was infected.

He came to the clinic to see if we could help him remove this condition. As Dr. Christopher stated, "There are no incurable diseases, just incurable patients". At the clinic we live by this statement.

We put him on the mucous-less diet along with the standard formulas of **Lower Bowel, Liver and Gallbladder** and later the **Blood Stream** formula. We also directly treated his lungs using the **Lung and Bronchial** and **Complete Tissue and Bone formulas**. He also did the three day cleanse using carrot juice. We put him on a strong regimen of garlic to combat the latent bacteria.

After being on the cleansing diet and the formulas for three months we had him tested again and the results showed no signs of the tuberculosis bacteria. I told him to hold on to that lab as proof for the future.

16.3 Steve – Chronic Pneumonia/Bronchitis

Here is a case with a patient who had been suffering from a long term chronic case of bronchitis with multiple instances of pneumonia each year. This had been going on for about ten years. He had to keep a rescue inhaler with him at all times and was on strong bronchial pharmaceuticals. He was also was a chronic smoker and stated he was not able to stop.

As in other cases, we placed him on the mucous-less diet, of which he only partially followed. I stated the most important dietary change had to be a complete lack of any kind of dairy. This he was able to do.

We followed the standard recommended protocol from Dr. Christopher and had him start on the formulas **Lower Bowel, Liver and Gallbladder**, **Lung and Bronchial** and the **Complete Tissue and Bone** capsules. Later in the program we added the **Blood Stream** formula.

Over time he noticed that a significant amount of mucous began to expectorate from his lungs. The original color was very dark, almost black. As the program progressed the color changed to a green, then a lighter yellow to eventually clear. His breathing continued to improve and he was able to stop taking his respiratory medications along with the rescue inhaler. He was still smoking but had cut it down to half. In time he was able to quite smoking altogether.

When he started the program he could not hold down a job. After about six months his health had improved enough to where he was able to go back to his construction job. He works there to this day.

CHAPTER 17

Chronic

17.1 Ruth – Lyme Disease

One of the joys we get at the clinic is the opportunity to be one of the only Lyme-literate clinics in Northern California. It is a sad state to find how little is known about this disease and how poorly the CDC encourages information. It is terribly under reported due to the CDC requirements being absurdly high for what can be classified as Lyme disease. Fortunately we have Dr. Christopher's knowledge and that of Dr. Burascano, the worlds leading authority on Lyme Disease. He is also very open to alternative medicine as an option for treatment. He has treated over 11,000 patients worldwide.

Ruth is a common example of a patient with Lyme Disease. Rarely does the patient receive treatment shortly after being bitten by the deer tick as this creature is quite small and most patients will not even realize they have been bitten. In only 20% of the cases does the classic "target" rash show up. In her case she was not diagnosed until about nine years after he initial infection. This results in what we classify as chronic or late term Lyme Disease with secondary infections.

This usually results in chronic joint and muscle pain, fatigue, a suppressed immune system along with a variety of other symptoms. She had been constantly misdiagnosed and was usually labeled with Chronic Fatigue Syndrome, a blanket diagnosis meaning they have no idea what is happening to the patient.

In her case we finally received a blood test back called the Western Blot Test. It showed the bacteria markers for the Lyme Disease organism. We began treatment immediately. One of the most important things to do for chronic Lyme Disease is to deal with the long term damage which is usually with the nerves. We also have to be careful treating the disorder too aggressively as a large die-off of the bacteria can actually harm the patient.

We started with the three day cleanse using carrot juice and afterwards she adopted the mucous-less diet. The cleansing formulas **Lower Bowel** and **Liver and Gallbladder** along with the **Kidney** formula were also utilized.

To aid in the nerve and joint damage we also added the formulas **MindTrac, Relax-Eze, St. John's Wort, Complete Tissue and Bone** and the **Joint** formula. To aid in the compromised immune system we added the **Adrenal** Formula with **Immucalm**.

Within the first month on the program she noticed an increased energy and a lessening of the joint and muscle pain. Her physician in her area has asked for us to consult with him so he can better treat his other patients with this issue.

While this program usually takes about a year to complete she continues to improve to this day.

For those interested, we have a book published with Amazon titled *A Holistic Approach to Healing Lyme Disease*.

17.2 Peggy – 92 prescription pills a week

Again we return to my wife Peggy. When we first got married I can say she loved me, just did not trust me with her health. She had been raised in the deep south where they tend to put physicians on a very high pedestal. This lasted for the first ten years of our marriage.

When we married she was on 92 prescription pills a week along with hip injects for a variety of different issues. She had extreme allergies to pollen and trees. She also had a very significant hormonal imbalance which left her in the fetal position every 28 days on the floor due to the pain of her periods. Her last condition was hypothyroidism, something they are told cannot be cured. She never did find relief from the pain or discomfort of any of her conditions while following conventional medicine.

After years of going to her physician she was told they give up and will schedule her for a full hysterectomy. The physician told her she was 36 years old and no longer needed her female organs. My wife had been with me long enough to know this was not a viable option. There are over 200,000 hysterectomies done in the United States each year and I do not believe any are necessary.

My wife had enough and asked me for help. I was overjoyed as I did not like seeing her in pain every 28 days. She was already a vegetarian so we cleaned her diet up a bit more and we started the program using **Lower Bowel**, **Liver and Gallbladder** and the **Blood Stream** as the cleansing components of the program.

For the allergies she started taking **Sinus-Plus** along with **Immucalm** and within a week her allergies were much improved. To this day she has never had the severe allergies from those days. Whenever a light attack occurs she simply takes a little **Immucalm** and **Sinus-Plus** again for a few days.

The hormonal imbalance required the use of the formulas **Female Reproductive**, **Hormonal Changese** along with Wheatgerm oil. She also started drinking about a quart of Red Raspberry tea a day.

The first 28 days rolled by and up came her first period on the program. While the pain was still quite severe she noted that it was somewhat less in intensity. All in all, it took about three months before she was able to happily declare she had her first normal period in life, in more than 20 years.

At this point now she was down from 92 prescription pills a week to just seven, for the thyroid. She was no longer having any hip injections. I asked her if she was ready to get rid of the hypothyroidism. The answer was a resounding yes.

For this issue it is important to feed and care for the Thyroid. We do this through the use of the formulas **Herbal Thyroid**, **Thyroid Maintenance** and **Kelp**. Mullein and Lobelia is also taken internally as a great glandular aid. During the later stages of the program we put a fomentation of the Mullein and Lobelia over the thyroid on her throat every evening before bed for six nights. It took another three months before she was off the last of the pills. It was getting close to the end of the year by this point so she decided to have a full blood panel done up by her old physician after the first of the year to see how she was doing.

When the results came back she was very pleased. It showed no sign of the allergies, hormonal imbalances or the hypothyroidism. Her physician looked at her and stated, in first person, "I guess I cured you". My wife walked out of there and never looked back.

A side note: 18 years later my wife entered menopause. Because she had already gotten her hormones in balance, menopause was not what most women in this country experience. There were no hot flashes, night sweats, changes in libido or vaginal dryness. Menopause is a gift meant to take a women from one phase of life to a more freer one. Unfortunately, most women in this country experience just the opposite.

17.3 Christine – High Blood Pressure

High blood pressure is epidemic in this country with prescription medication for it one of the highest recommended. We had a patient by the name of Christine who was on two of these types of drugs and was beginning to show liver issues. Even while on the medication her blood pressure remained constantly high.

We put her on the standard program with dietary changes, the three day cleanse and the cleansing formulas **Lower Bowel**, **Liver and Gallbladder** and **Blood Stream**. To aid the blood pressure issue directly we recommended the formulas **Hawthorne Berry Syrup** and **Blood Circulation**.

Within the first month her blood pressure began to drop to the normal range while still on her pharmaceuticals. By month two her blood pressure was beginning to drop still further and her other primary had to drop her dosage of the drugs, By month three her physician had to completely take her off of them as her blood pressure was dropping too low. Off the drugs her blood pressure was now within the normal range and we were able to take her off of ours and to this day she is on none of the previous drugs.

17.4 Susan – High Cholesterol/Triglycerides

Susan had one of the highest triglyceride levels I had ever seen. She was in the danger zone being around 2000 when the average patient should be no higher than 150. She loved her sweets and carbs and seafood. Her cholesterol was also very elevated.

As always, we recommended the dietary changes utilizing the three day cleanse with the mucous-less diet. The usual cleansing formulas were also incorporated. The **Blood Stream** formula was also very significant here as it helped clean her blood out as an aid to clear out some of the cholesterol. We added garlic and flax and kelp as well to drop these levels further.

We ran the usual labs to monitor her levels and for a while they did drop some but very slowly. One of things that can confuse a patient is when they get on a vegan diet and find that their cholesterol continues to rise. This can be from two basic issues. One is that the liver is most likely damaged and need some assist. Also, during one's lifetime, when the liver cannot detoxify enough of the poisons traveling through the body, it will basically "take a bullet" for you and store them.

When you go on a good cleansing diet the liver suddenly finds itself in a large supply of the needed nutrients to do the job and it will attempt to convert this backlog. This can come out as bile and quite a bit of damaged cholesterol or LDL. I always tell the patients that if they can be patient the levels will eventually drop.

To further aid this issue we added milk thistle to heal the liver from a lifetime of bad choices. Within about three months the liver had healed enough to drop her triglycerides levels to 600 and by the fifth month she came back with a clean bill of health. She was no longer in danger of liver or heart disease.

17.5 Jack – Near Sighted

It is always a pleasure to see a patient relieved of a crutch that they have been hanging on to for most of their life. Glasses are no exception to this rule.

Jack had been wearing glasses for many years and was ready to let them go. We had already been treating his daughter for a serious hormonal imbalance due to endometriosis at the age of 27 and then a hysterectomy so he was familiar with the program.

While he did not follow the program very well he still ended up with wonderful results. He barely made any dietary changes though he did try and stay away from dairy. He used the **Lower Bowel** and the **Liver and Gallbladder** formulas and added the formula **Herbal Eyebright** to his regimen. He used it twice a day externally and also used it internally.

Two months passed after using the formulas consistently he decided to go back to the DMV to take an eye test. He passed the test and the DMV removed the restriction from his license.

17.6 Virgil – Shingles and Heart Blockage

Here I get to return to a family member for a case history. This time it was for my father in law Virgil. When my wife and I married I was the foreigner (not from Alabama) who had come to take their daughter away from them. Needless to say, I was not well loved in that family.

About ten years into our marriage my wife and I opened our first clinic. Sometime after this Virgil called us and asked for help. Without us knowing it, he had been suffering from a very serious case of Shingles. This had been going on for about six weeks. His physician had to admit to him that he did not know what to do for him and asked if he knew of any old family remedies. It was at this time Virgil called us.

We immediately drove out to their house and found a man in such pain and misery. He was covered with the lesions from the top of his head and down his back and legs. We treated the shingles both topically and orally. Topically, we treated him with our formula called **Herbadyne** using Myrrh, Goldenseal and Cayenne. Internally, we treated him with high doses of Echinacea and Goldenseal root. Goldenseal is a wonderful antiviral. The dosage was five capsules five times a day.

By the next morning he called us and reported the pain was already diminishing and within a week the shingle's lesions were gone. I went from being the black sheep of the family to them going around church bragging about their son in law the doctor.

Two years later he called us again over another issue. His cardiologist found a 90% heart block and recommended open heart surgery. Virgil asked for a three month reprieve to try something different. The physician consented.

We knew he would not change his diet so we recommended a simply routine of distilled water and apple cider vinegar. This utilized mixing a glass of distilled water with a tablespoon or more of apple cider vinegar.

This was to be drank four times a day, six days a week. He was to follow this for the full three months.

After three months he went back to the physician and they canceled the surgery as the heart blockage went from 90% to 0%. He also experienced an interesting side effect from this program.

Before he stated the apple cider vinegar cleanse he had been unable to perform sexually for about 15 years. He happily reported that all systems were functioning once the vinegar had cleansed out all of the arteries.

17.7 Betsy – Heavy Metal Toxicity

One of the most prevalent conditions in America today as well as in other industrialized nations is heavy metal toxicity. It is found in the food, the air, the soil, cigarette smoking and in the cloths we wear. Pharmaceuticals are filled with them such as mercury, aluminum, cadmium, lead and arsenic.

Some time back a 47 year old female patient came into our clinic complaining of a number of autoimmune type reactions as well as a serious candida and mold infection. During her intake we found that she was a potter and sculptor who made extensive use of glazing. Heavy metals can be found in the clay itself as well as the chemicals used for glazing. Her home also had a very serious mold problem. Her blood work showed infections and a hair analysis showed extensive heavy metals as can be seen by the following lab result:

TOXIC METALS		RESULT µg/g	REFERENCE INTERVAL	PERCENTILE 68th 95th
Aluminum	(Al)	8.1	< 7.0	
Antimony	(Sb)	0.12	< 0.050	
Arsenic	(As)	0.048	< 0.060	
Barium	(Ba)	4.0	< 2.0	
Beryllium	(Be)	< 0.01	< 0.020	
Bismuth	(Bi)	0.096	< 2.0	
Cadmium	(Cd)	0.12	< 0.050	
Lead	(Pb)	5.6	< 0.60	
Mercury	(Hg)	0.15	< 0.80	
Platinum	(Pt)	< 0.003	< 0.005	
Thallium	(Tl)	< 0.001	< 0.002	
Thorium	(Th)	0.002	< 0.002	
Uranium	(U)	0.014	< 0.060	
Nickel	(Ni)	0.29	< 0.30	
Silver	(Ag)	5.5	< 0.15	
Tin	(Sn)	1.1	< 0.30	
Titanium	(Ti)	0.57	< 0.70	
Total Toxic Representation				

She was very high in Antimony, Barium, Lead, Nickel and Silver. These metals are notorious for wiping out the intestinal flora and bringing bout a severe candida overgrowth, thereby compromising the immune system. This left her open to so many other co-infections such as mold and other bacterial types. Her original presenting complaints included candida and hormonal imbalances.

We stated her off with our standard candida cleanse, mentioned earlier in this document. This utilized a vegan diet due to it's low inflammatory nature and one low in natural sugar. She had to avoid all sugars and alcohol, even fruits for at least 18 days as well as use holistic medications for killing the candida, such as Black walnut and Pau'd Arco. We keep the bowels moving to help eliminate the dead yeast.

By the end of the 18 days she noticed a marked improvement in her thinking and level of energy. She proceeded to have the home cleaned out from the mold while we treated her for the mold in lungs, again, using the above mold and yeast formulas, but at a much lower dosage and for several months. She remained on the vegan diet as it is well established that the fiber and anti-oxidants and other chemicals in the plants help chelate the heavy metals from her body.

At this time we also prescribed a natural heavy metal formula called Dr. Christopher's Bugle Heavy Metal Formula. It utilizes Bugleweed, a known herb with a very strong history of success for removing heavy metals from the body. She remained on this program for at least six months. As each month passed on the program she felt her health improving which we conformed with blood work demonstrating the infections were disappearing. We finally ran another heavy metal hair test six months later. The surprising results are shown below:

		RESULT µg/g	REFERENCE INTERVAL	PERCENTILE 68th 95th
\multicolumn{5}{|c|}{TOXIC METALS}				
Aluminum	(Al)	3.6	< 7.0	
Antimony	(Sb)	0.035	< 0.050	
Arsenic	(As)	0.048	< 0.060	
Barium	(Ba)	1.5	< 2.0	
Beryllium	(Be)	< 0.01	< 0.020	
Bismuth	(Bi)	0.013	< 2.0	
Cadmium	(Cd)	0.046	< 0.050	
Lead	(Pb)	1.2	< 0.60	
Mercury	(Hg)	0.08	< 0.80	
Platinum	(Pt)	< 0.003	< 0.005	
Thallium	(Tl)	< 0.001	< 0.002	
Thorium	(Th)	0.001	< 0.002	
Uranium	(U)	0.020	< 0.060	
Nickel	(Ni)	0.12	< 0.30	
Silver	(Ag)	1.4	< 0.15	
Tin	(Sn)	0.14	< 0.30	
Titanium	(Ti)	0.34	< 0.70	
Total Toxic Representation				

As you can see from the above lab, the heavy metals showed a marked improvement which was mirrored in her improved energy levels, thinking and memory abilities and a total lack of bronchial and sinus issues.

She remains vegan to this day and is a shining example of a healthy and happy individual. We are all very proud of her.

CHAPTER 18

Incurables

18.1 Lilly – Utecarea

According to Wikipedia:

Urticaria (from the Latin *urtica* , "nettle" from *urere*, "to burn"), commonly referred to as **hives**, is a kind of skin rash notable for pale red, raised, itchy bumps. Hives may cause a burning or stinging sensation. They are frequently caused by allergic reactions; however, there are many nonallergic causes. Most cases of hives lasting less than six weeks (acute urticaria) are the result of an allergic trigger. Chronic urticaria (hives lasting longer than six weeks) is rarely due to an allergy.
The majority of chronic hives cases have an unknown (idiopathic) cause. In perhaps as many as 30–40% of patients with chronic idiopathic urticaria, it is caused by an autoimmune reaction.

In all of my career I have only had one patient with this condition. She was a 60 year old women with severe hives from the top of her head to the bottom of her feet. When she first came to the clinic all she could do was squirm in her chair while she related her story. It broke my heart to see her suffering so much. All the conventional medical establishment could do was to give her Prednisone.

Since it is an autoimmune condition we recommended the Incurables program from Dr. Christopher. She immediately did the three day cleanse using carrot juice and started on the mucous-less diet. All dairy and other animal products were removed from her diet and more raw food was added. After the cleanse she began taking the cleansing formulas **Lower Bowel**, **Liver and Gallbladder** and two months in she started on the **Blood Stream**. We rarely use the **Blood Stream** at the start of the program as we do not want to send too much to the liver until it has been strengthened by the formula **Liver and Gallbladder**.

We also stated her on the **Immucalm** formula which calmed her immune system down while still keeping it strong. This had the immediate result on diminishing the number of hives she was experiencing each day. She also used a salve we made from Comfrey, Plantain and Chickweed for soothing and healing the tender skin.

Because of the diet and the cleansing formulas with the **Immucalm**, the issue faded until all of her hives vanished. She has now moved forward with her learning and has just graduated from the Family Herbalist course at our clinic. She will make a wonderful herbalist in her home.

By the way, her family originally intervened to stop her from taking our treatments but now are so happy with the results they have put her back to work.

18.2 Betty – Multiple Sclerosis

As one of the most devastating illnesses we have dealt with at the clinic, we have also been overjoyed to see the amount of success using Dr. Christopher's protocols. Betty was a 33 year women who came into the clinic with advanced M.S. She was already dependent on a cane and her eyesight and voice were being affected. Her MRI showed three lesions on her brain and the prognosis was a long term progression towards a wheel chair.

As with all of these types of illnesses we prefer to follow Dr. Christopher's Incurables protocols. We presented her with the plan and she threw herself into the program. After the three day cleanse with carrot juice she immediately went vegan and quickly changed her diet over to about 80% raw, using mainly fresh fruits and vegetables. She also started the cleansing formulas of **Lower Bowel, Liver and Gallbladder** and the **Blood Stream** formula after two months.

To directly combat the M.S. she also starting taking the formulas **Immucalm**, **Relax-Eze** and the **Ear and Nerve**. As we stated before, due to this being an autoimmune issue, **Immucalm** calmed her immune system while allowing it to remain strong. While **Immucalm** does not cure M.S. every program should contain two prongs, one as a curative and the other as a palliative. The palliative is simply meant to make the patient comfortable while waiting for the cure to take effect. **Immucalm** allows the body to slow or stop the damage to the nervous system while the other formulas and diet are allowed to heal.

The formula **Relax-Eze** aids the body in calming and feeding the nervous system. The **Ear and Nerve** formula has been shown to be an excellent aid in healing the nerves and assisting with balance. She would use the **Ear and Nerve** each night in her ears before bed as well as taking it internally.

After just three weeks on the program she was able to put her cane away. As the months progressed, her balance improved to the point where she could wear high heals and was able to move out of her parents house for the first time in her life. She now holds down a job and is doing very well.

An UPDATE:

Recently, I have been performing reflexology treatments on Betty and with just three treatments to date she is already showing further improvement. Circulation is improving and what little numbness remained in her feet is completely disappearing.

An interesting side note is that we are finding in more and more cases that this issue as well as many others such as Lupus, RA, ALS, Parkensen's and many others are actually Lyme disease misdiagnosed. Please make sure to ask your doctor for further testing before you accept one of the above type of verdicts.

For those interested, we have a book published with Amazon titled *A Holistic Approach to Healing Lyme Disease.*

18.3 Matthew – Sigmoid Cancer

Matthew had been suffering with a Sigmoid tumor since 2009 and had already undergone one surgery for it as well as radiation. The radiation had destroyed his bladder and he was now using an external bag for the urine. Sadly, the cancer returned. Each year he had to receive a cat-scan and an MRI to watch the progression of the disease.

In 2013 he came into the clinic looking for an alternative solution to the medical industries drugs and radiation. He was somewhat reluctant to change his diet but we made it very clear that without a diet change, an issue of this manner would not be cured. He agreed and we began the program.

As with all cases such as this, he started with the three day cleanse using carrot juice. Carrot juice is one of the main juices to be used during any cancer program. Mixed with beet juice it is an excellent liver cleanser. We also started him immediately on the **Lower Bowel** as the cancer was in that area. 100% of the time cancer always starts in the bowels and is aggravated by a poorly functioning liver. The **Liver and Gallbladder** formula was also added.

While we normally only keep patients on the **Lower Bowel** and **Liver and Gallbladder** for three months total and the **Blood Stream** for one month at the end of the cleansing, in Matthew's case we kept him on the **Lower Bowel** and the **Blood Stream** formulas for most of the program. The reason for this is that cancer is always a condition of the bowels and therefore we wanted to keep the cleansing and healing properties of the **Lower Bowel** working the entire time. The **Blood Stream** was to aid in cleansing the blood of the cancer. While it was a cancer of the colon, the blood stream is always involved.

All of our cancer programs range from nine months to a year. This is to insure that the cancer has been eradicated. By the tenth month it came time for Matthew's yearly cat-scan and MRI. The good news came that there was no sign of the cancer spreading as seen from the cat-scan.

The MRI was inclusive to whether it could see any cancer. A final urine test was performed one year after we started the program and it came back negative. The colon cancer was gone.

Matthew of course was overjoyed as was I. It is very moving to see a patient recover from cancer without any more of the body being destroyed due to chemo and radiation therapies. He stated that he felt "normal" again for the first time in years.

18.4 Stacy – Polycystic Ovarian Syndrome

Polycystic Ovarian Syndrome affects approximately one out of fifteen women in the U.S. each year. As described in Wiki:

Polycystic ovary syndrome (PCOS), also called **hyperandrogenic anovulation (HA)**, or **Stein–Leventhal syndrome**, is a set of symptoms due to a hormone imbalance in women. Symptoms include: irregular or no menstrual periods, heavy periods, excess body and facial hair, acne, pelvic pain, trouble getting pregnant, and patches of thick, darker, velvety skin. Associated conditions include: type 2 diabetes, obesity, obstructive sleep apnea, heart disease, mood disorders, and endometrial cancer.

PCOS is due to a combination of genetic and environmental factors. Risk factors include obesity, not enough physical exercise, and a family history of someone with the condition. Diagnosis is based on two of the following three findings: no ovulation, high androgen levels, and ovarian cysts. Cysts may be detectable by ultrasound. Other conditions that produce similar symptoms include adrenal hyperplasia, hypothyroidism, and hyperprolactinemia.

PCOS has no cure. Treatment may involve lifestyle changes such as weight loss and exercise. Birth control pills may help with improving the regularity of periods, excess hair, and acne. Metformin and anti-androgens may also help. Other typical acne treatments and hair removal techniques may be used. Efforts to improve fertility include weight loss, clomiphene, or metformin. In vitro fertilization is used by some in whom other measures are not effective.

You will notice that it states there is no cure. The standard treatment plan is purely allopathic and uses birth control pills, which puts the woman at an increased risk of breast cancer. We are happy to report that Dr. Christopher was correct when he stated there is no incurable disease, only incurable people. Our case history here is about a patient of ours by the name of Stacy, who had, past tense, Polycystic Ovarian Syndrome, PCOS for short.

She came to our clinic at the age of 25 with a serious hormonal imbalance and excess hair growth.. She was also overweight and could not lose the extra pounds.

We ran the standard saliva and blood tests and it showed she had PCOS. Her previous physician had told her there was nothing she could do but take birth control pills to alleviate the symptoms, which did not work.

We put her on the standard program of **Lower Bowel**, and **Liver and Gallbladder** with the **Blood Stream** formula introduced later. She also started with a three day cleanse using carrot juice. She did notice a significant cleanse reaction of headaches and nausea while undergoing the cleanse.

To aid in the hormonal imbalance we started her on the formulas **Female Reproductive**, **Hormonal Changese**, wheatgerm oil and at least a quart of Red Raspberry tea each day, six days a week, one day off.

One of her other main complaints was Interstitial Cystitis, an inflammation of the lining of the bladder. For this she took the **Kidney** and **Bladder** formulas along with the **Soothing Digestion** combination. Within a week she began to notice the pain in her bladder was lessening. Overtime, this completely vanished.

We had to wait for her next cycle to occur but the good news came that it was somewhat better, with less pain and flow. Over the next three months her period completely normalized for the first time in her life.

One special note is that during this process she strictly followed the mucous-less diet and has to this day remained mostly raw. We have since run the same labs as before and her blood and saliva work shows no sign of the PCOS. An added benefit is that with all PCOS cases there is a serious issue with insulin resistance, hence making it difficult to lose the weight. For her, the insulin resistance completely disappeared and she has loss around forty pounds.

There is no such thing as an incurable disease...

18.5 James – Psoriasis/Genetic Issues

We have always considered James as one of our most special and well loved patients. He came to the clinic with one of the worst cases of psoriasis I have ever seen and was also afflicted with functional autism at the age of 35.

Below is an example of the stomach and back before we started treatment:

3 Jul 2013

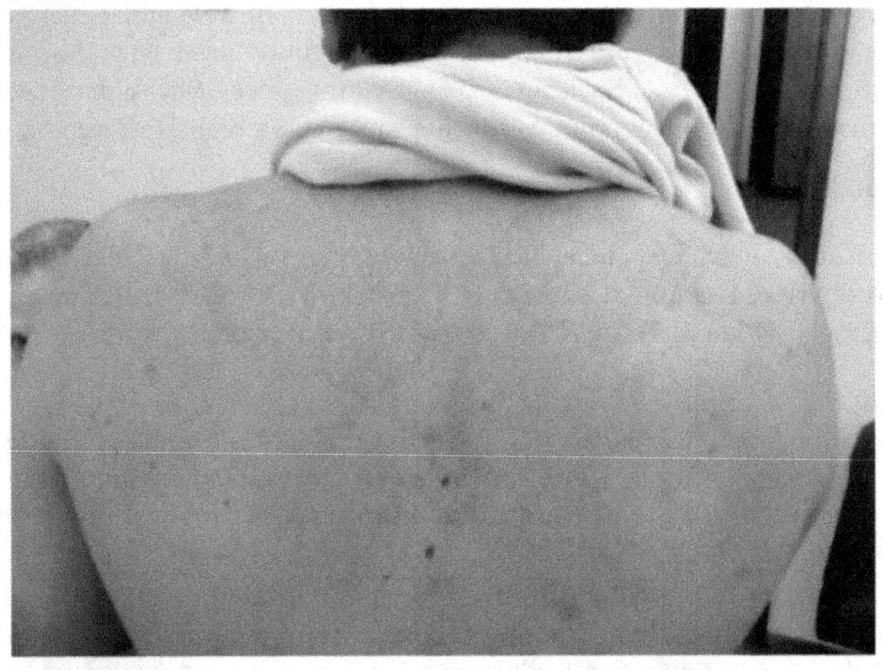

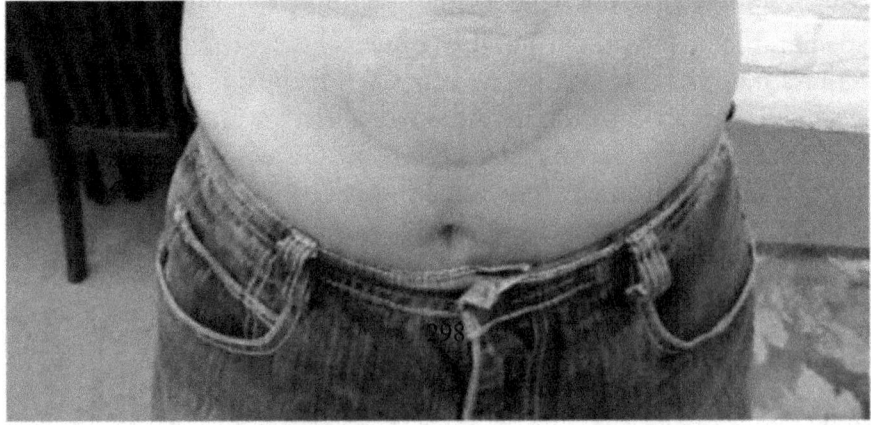

At first we mainly focused on the psoriasis and this is what his father had requested. Because this condition is an auto-immune disorder, we requested that James strictly follow the mucous-less diet. He did so wonderfully. Of all the patients who have crossed ours doors, he was the most accepting of the diet and never once complained. One of the things we do at the clinic is to supply our patients with a variety of sample menu plans and will even bring food into the clinic for them to try. This has been a great success as most folks are very nervous about changing their diets and have no idea where to start. By instructing them and taking time to teach, it can remove a significant amount of stress from the program.

We also recommended using the formulas **Lower Bowel**, **Liver and Gallbladder** and **Blood Stream.** You may notice that no matter what the condition or issue may be, there is a common vein found in all of them. This is the use of the cleansing formulas just listed above. Hippocrates stated to cleanse and nourish and Dr. Christopher taught us this as well. It has proven true time and again that if the body is cleansed it will uptake nutrients and natural medicines much faster. It is safe to say that 95% of all patients go through the three day cleanse and follow up using these formulas.

To work directly with the psoriasis we added the formulas **Complete Tissue and Bone** and **Immucalm**. Again, **Immucalm** calms the immune system while keeping it strong which helped slow the progress of the disease while the rest of the program worked on healing it.

Very quickly we began to notice a diminishing of the scales on his body. The itching vanished as well. But after about four months the progress came to a halt. The scales remained at a certain level and nothing I did seemed to aid the situation.

One day while James and his father were in the clinic we spoke about his disposition. His work place had complained about James's attitude and aggressive behaviors and had threatened to remove him from the county program. I knew that stress and emotions can have a serious affect on psoriasis so we ran a urinalysis for neurotransmitters. We had seen in the past that children with autism had a serious imbalance within the chemicals of the brain. The test came back very conclusive with indications of a propensity towards aggression and OCD (Obsessive Compulsive Disorder).

At this point we immediately went to work on the brain. We recommended the formulas **St. John's Wort**, **Relax-Eze** and **MindTrac**. We have seen amazing results with **St. John's Wort** as most patients in this condition have a serotonin imbalance. **St. John's Wort** works beautifully.

Relax-Eze calmed the nerves while feeding the brain. **MindTrac** worked specifically on the neurotransmitters. After just one month on this new regimen we ran another urinalysis for the neurotransmitters. The results were astounding. Every single neurotransmitter began to move towards the healthy range.

It was also at this time that we saw the greatest improvement in his psoriasis. Within a couple of months many of the spots completely disappeared with the rest showing a wonderful improvement.

Below is a recent picture of one of the worse spots he had originally displayed:

18 Mar 2015

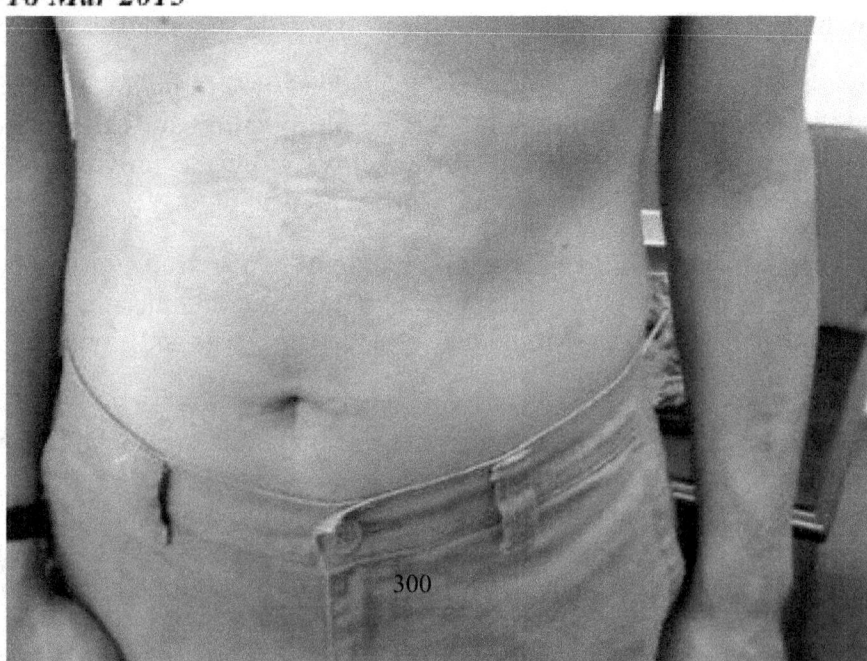

18.6 Robert – Type 1 Diabetes

Robert was a 35 year old patient with type 1 diabetes. This is the type considered incurable due to it's auto-immune character. He was morbidly obese weighing 362 pounds when he started the program. He also exhibited extensive foot neuropathy with severe skin abrasions due to the lack of healing. The nerves had died within the feet which made them feel like he was walking on blocks of wood. All his past healthcare providers had given up on him and claimed there was no hope. The disease would progress to the point where he would begin to lose his feet.

As with all patients we informed him there is no such thing as an incurable disease. He needed to take responsibility for his illness and to be a part of the cure. All any healthcare provider can do is to guide or teach the patient and to support them during the treatments. The cure is between the patient and what they believe in as a higher power.

As with all patients of this type of condition, he did the three cleanse with carrot juice and switched to the mucous-less diet. **Lower Bowel**, **Liver and Gallbladder** , **Blood Stream** and the **Kidney** formulas were incorporated into his daily regimen for six days a week with a day off and then repeat for months. We also added the **Pancreas** and **Immucalm** formulas to directly work with the condition.

All patients who follow the incurables program are informed this could take from nine months to a year to compete but that they should see some results within the first month. This was a wonderful example of that truth. Within the first three weeks on the program his amount of insulin used each day was cut in half and his blood sugar began to stabilize.

He was also able to report to his other primary a new and unexpected change. Never in his life had he seen any progress in slowing the disease. When he returned to his previous primary after six weeks she was shocked to find that the wounds were healing and that he was beginning to have feeling return to his feet. She quickly encouraged him to continue. He had lost approximately thirty pounds in that same period.

This type of progress continued until he was ready to take control of the disease and to manage it himself.

18.7 Nancy – Myasthenia Gravis

According to Wiki:

Myasthenia gravis (from Greek μύς "muscle", ἀσθένεια "weakness", and Latin: *gravis* "serious"; abbreviated **MG**) is either an autoimmune or congenital neuromuscular disease that leads to fluctuating muscle weakness and fatigue. In the most common cases, muscle weakness is caused by circulating antibodies that block acetylcholine receptors at the postsynaptic neuromuscular junction, inhibiting the excitatory effects of the neurotransmitter acetylcholine on nicotinic receptors at neuromuscular junctions. Alternatively, in a much rarer form, muscle weakness is caused by a genetic defect in some portion of the neuromuscular junction, that is inherited at birth as opposed to developing it through autoimmunity later in life or through passive transmission by the mother's immune system at birth.

Myasthenia is treated medically with acetylcholinesterase inhibitors or immunosuppressants, and, in selected cases, thymectomy. The disease is diagnosed in 3 to 30 people per million per year. Diagnosis is becoming more common due to increased awareness. MG must be distinguished from congenital myasthenic syndromes that can present similar symptoms but do not respond to immunosuppressive treatments.

As you may notice, here again, this is considered incurable and is treated usually through immunosuppressants. These types of drugs leave the patient open to every bacteria, virus or fungus they may come into contact. The conventional medical community also perform a very serious surgery called thymectomy, where they remove the Thymus gland, one of the most important immune glands.

They perform these surgeries and prescribe these drugs because of the way they look at the auto-immune disease. They believe the body's immune system has lost control and begins to attack the body.

We do not believe this philosophy. We believe the immune system is working perfectly. In every type of auto-immune condition a particular cell type in the body is in a weaken state and does not display it's marker or flag which informs the immune system that it is part of self. The immune system therefore destroys the cell. Our protocol is to support the immune system while calming it down aiding the body in regrowing cells with the proper markers.

Our patient in this case was Nancy, a 34 year old woman with MG. She came to my attention right after graduating from the School of Natural Healing. I had turned in my financial paperwork to my CPA and Nancy was her secretary. When Nancy saw my paperwork and realized I was a natural, holistic healthcare provider she gave me a call. I informed her that I had just graduated but I would not turn her away. At that point we had not opened our first clinic. She was still willing, due to desperation, to see me. To protect ourselves legally, we opened our very first clinic to give us some type of umbrella with which to treat her. So I now had my first patient and she was of the most dangerous types of this condition.

During her first visit she asked for an exam to show us the scar from the thymectomy. She was also on Imuran and Prednisone and was told she would be on these for the rest of her life. She was also informed that the thymectomy failed and that she could have an MG crisis at any time. An MG crisis is when the patient attempts to breath but the signal is not received at the diaphragm.

As with any patient with the classic incurable tag, I inform them that they will be looking at a nine month to a year program. She would also be required to go on the mucous-less diet with a progression towards a significant portion of it being raw. The three day cleanse was also recommended.

With good faith she completed the cleanse and began the diet. She started on the basic formulas **Lower Bowel**, **Liver and Gallbladder**, **Blood Stream** and **Kidney**. We also added the formulas **Immuncalm**, **Complete Tissue and Bone** and **Ear and Nerve**. The **Complete Tissue and Bone** was added to aid in rebuilding the muscle and nerve tissues while the **Ear and Nerve** was very specific to the nerve regrowth. **Relax-Eze** was also added for nerve regrowth and to calm them.

She never did have an MG crisis during the program, which for her only lasted nine months. Due to her age she was able to heal more quickly than some of the older patients. In that short period of time she was able to get off of the Imuran and Prednisone.

Sixteen years ago I could not do the lab work I can today so I recommended she return to her previous primary and get a series of labs done to see what her present condition might show. When the labs were completed her physician looked at her with a stunned looked on his face and remarked that she must be in remission. To him she could not possibly be cured. At this point I told her she was through with the program and to simply watch her diet and follow healthy lifestyle choices.

We kept the clinic open for some time before we moved toward the west coast. Seven years past when I received a letter from the IRS claiming a $200 error on my taxes from back in the days when I was using my old CPA. I got on the phone and called her and to my great joy Nancy answered the phone.

We are very informal at our clinic and we are all on a first name basis. I happily exclaimed Nancy and she responded with yelling Earendil. I asked how she was doing after seven years and she proudly informed me that the disease never did return.

This is the reason I do what I do.

18.8 Cathy – Epstein Barr

One of the most common disorders in this society is chronic fatigue syndrome. It is usually caused by either a serious Candida overgrowth or by an Epstein Barr viral infection. It is also considered incurable. Most physicians will not even test for it because they feel it is a waste of time to check for something they cannot "fix".

Cathy was a 55 year old woman with confirmed Epstein Barr. This brought on extensive fatigue to the point she had difficulty getting out of bed before 10:00 or 11:00 in the morning. This caused a significant amount of stress as she ran her own business and this impacted her ability to perform the basic tasks the work required. It also caused muscle and joint pain similar to arthritis.

She completed the three day cleanse using apple juice and switched to a vegan diet. We also started her on **Lower Bowel, Liver and Gallbladder** and later, **Blood Stream**. To directly combat the virus we recommended significant doses of Garlic along with Echinacea and Goldenseal. **Immucalm** was added to calm her immune system. The **Joint** formula was also used as an aid for the joint and muscle pains.

Within the first month she began to notice she had a little bit more energy and was not sleeping as late. Her joint pain also began to diminish. Within a total of six months all of the fatigue had vanished and she was awakening refreshed by 5:00 or 6:00 in the morning. We ran a final Epstein Barr blood test and it came back negative.

I still see her running her company for the various grocery stores in our area and she always has a smile on her face.

18.9 Carol – Hysterectomy at age 27

Currently in the United States there are approximately 200,000 hysterectomies a year and I would be willing to say that is about 200,000 too many. One of the most memorable cases was a young lady who came to us at the age of 27.

She had been suffering from endometriosis and her other doctor had already had one ovary removed and was pushing for the other, along with her uterus and cervix. Her parents knew me and tried to get her to come into the clinic before the final surgery. Alas, they did not convince her and she went ahead and had everything else removed.

She eventually did come to the clinic as a patient but this was three months post-OP and 5 foot five inches and 85 pounds, pale as a sheet and addicted to Vicodin the pain killer prescribed for after surgery care. She was in tears as she felt no one would care to marry her since she could not have children and the previous doctor had told her she would have to wear an Estrogen patch the rest of her life. Needless to say there was little I could do to help with the baby issue but I told her she would be able to avoid the hormone replacement therapy. She was skeptical as she believed all estrogen came form the ovaries but I explained to her that the liver was also capable of producing it if in a healthy state. She decided to give our program a try.

We ran a hormone panel before treatment which was able to give us a "before" snapshot of her state. She then changed her diet to a healthy vegan based one and did a candida cleanse to prepare her immune system. This also allowed her to better assimilate her foods and then medications we gave her. After it was completed we stated her on the same program as mentioned earlier with patients with PCOS using herbs such as Red Raspberry tea, Blessed Thistle, Ginseng, Licorice root, False Unicorn, Sarsaparilla and Black Cohosh. She also continued to do colon and liver cleanses as well.

Within three months she was back up to 110 pounds, brown skin and no longer on Vicodin. We ran a three month hormone panel and without any hormone replacement therapy her Estrogen, Progesterone and Testosterone were back up within the normal ranges. She no longer had to take any of our medications.

Follow ups showed she never did experience any of the normal menopausal symptoms for women who have had a complete hysterectomy. She was instructed to stay on a healthy, vegan diet and to continue to take her Red Raspberry Tea on a daily basis.

18.10 Samuel – Chronic system wide body rash

It is sad to me when a patient comes into the clinic after months or years of suffering due to the fact they were never properly diagnosed. Following is one such case.

Samuel was a 58 year old male who presented with a rash from his head to his feet and had been suffering from it for the past nine months. The previous three months before we had our first appointment he had spent sitting in a chair or in bed as any movement caused it to flare up into an intense, maddening itch. He had gone to doctor after doctor including specialists such as dermatologist and even had skin punch biopsies done, to no avail for a diagnosis. His quality of life was at an all-time low and he had lost hope for a cure.

I went over his intake form and did what any good doctor would do and that is to try and find the root cause, not just treat the symptoms. I inquired as to what may have happened or changed in his life about nine or ten months ago. The only thing he could think of is that he had his mercury fillings removed just before the rash appeared. He described the procedure the dentist used. I discussed with the patient that the wrong procedure was done and that the mercury vapor had been inhaled and swallowed during the dental office visit.

Ingesting or inhaling mercury is like taking a massive dose of an antibiotic. It will destroy your bacterial micro-flora and leave you open to a massive candida overgrowth. I told him the rash was Candida Vasculitis, very common after such an event.

As with all of our chronic patients, the first thing we do is the 18 day candida cleanse. As mentioned earlier, this utilize a healthy, non-inflammatory vegan diet with herbal medications such as Black Walnut and Pau'd Arco for eliminating the yeast. We also employ the use of Slippery Elm bark and Licorice root for soothing and healing the intestinal walls, so inflamed from the yeast overgrowth.

By the end of the 18 days, his body wide rash had shrunk to a small patch on his upper left arm. He stated he was feeling wonderful and his energy was much improved. I started him on a heavy metal detox using Dr. Christopher's Bugle Heavy Metal formula and he remained on the diet to allow his body a chance to heal while the chelation continued.

After a total of two months he no longer experienced any sign of the rashes and the detox was completed. He and his wife continued to be patients with the clinic for various other minor issues for a couple of years and the rash never made another appearance.

18.11 Kim – Inoperable colon/appendix cancer

The cancer rate statistics in the year 1900 was 1 out 50 would have this disease sometime in their lifetime. By the 1970's, the start of the "war on Cancer", the rate was up to 1 out of 10. Today it has grown to 1 out 2 people in the United States will experience cancer sometime in their lifetime. Needless to say, the war on cancer is not being won.

At our clinic we have seen many. Many cases of cancer and the number of patients presenting this illness is on the rise within our practice. One particular case stands out as one of my patients to have had the joy and privilege to know.

She was a 59 year old woman who originally came to the clinic to be treated for psoriasis. During her initial appointment she asked if I would check on lump on her lower right abdomen. I told her I would be happy to check. She stated her other doctor had checked and dismissed it as a simply fatty deposit but her heart told her different. When we were going over her treatment plan for the psoriasis I lead her and her husband into the exam room.

I have been around quite a bit of cancer in my 20+ years of practice and as soon as I palpated the area I knew what it was. But, I kept the traditional poker face and suggested we check with ultrasound. We have ultrasound at the clinic so it was a simple matter of setting the machine up and within five minutes we were scanning the site. Her entire abdominal cavity was full of what appeared to be tumors and acites (fluid filled pockets often caused by cancer in the bowels and appendix).

The poker face was gone and she could see there was some concern. I requested we get some blood work done to get a better idea. She agreed and when the lab results came in it confirmed a 95% likelihood of cancer. She became very upset with her doctor dismissing her since at this point she had lost two months of possible treatment time. She returned to them and showed them our results. At this point the other doctor panicked and reran all of my tests and found the same results. The final diagnosis was colon and appendix cancer with Pseudomyxoma peritonei (PMP) .She was staged at stage four.

Or course, the recommended treatment plan from them was to surgically bulk the cancer and to run a very risky chemo therapy treatment that requires extensive blood transfusions. As a Jehovah Witness she was not able to accept the treatment. The other doctors told her she would be dead in six months if she did not take the chemotherapy. She still refused and returned to our clinic for a holistic program.

As with all chronic patients, the first step was the candida cleanse. Again, this is done to aid in healing the immune system. Cancer is a systemic failure of the immune system and it is a well established fact that it is important for the patient's own immune system to begin to fight back. Normally, most people are exposed to cancer as tiny little errant cells. In a healthy immune system we respond to the threat and destroy the cancer cells on our own. In the case of cancer patients, their immune system was compromised and did not destroy the threat.

This can have a wide variety of root causes but in the end we ALWAYS and with no exceptions, find each cancer patient presenting extensive candida overgrowth. It is our job then, at the beginning, to aid the patient in reestablishing the intestinal environment. Once this is done than the patient has a higher likelihood of having a stronger immune system.

Once the 18 day candida cleanse is completed we then proceed with actually fighting the cancer. The patient remains on a vegan diet but at this point they begin to increase dramatically the percentage of raw, live food. We supply them with a wide variety of meal plans, recipes and nutrition charts so this does not become a boring diet.

We also being the holistic medication portion of the regimen. Colon and liver cleanses are done throughout the program along with herbal formulas utilizing Poke root, Red Raspberry tea, Milk thistle, blood cleanser formulas using Red Clover, and Thunder god vine root.

Thunder god vine root has been studied extensively out of China, Germany and even here in the states under Johns Hopkins University. Clinical trial studies seem to indicate that this herb out of China is able to begin the process of apoptosis with in 40 days. Apoptosis is the process by which cancer cells switch off their DNA and "commit suicide", so to speak.

With programs such as this kind, we ask the patient to return to the clinic once a month so we can check their progress, run vitals, run tests in house, all in an effort to monitor their treatments. We also regularly ran blood work on her cancer markers.

With each visit she reported feeling better and the masses, examined through ultrasound continued to shrink. Her cancer marker also continued to drop closer to the normal ranges. MRIs and CT scans were run about every six months.

At her last MRI scan along with ultrasound and blood work the local hospital declared no sign of the cancer any longer and to their surprise, her colon had "rebuilt itself".

Something we try and teach each patient is that he body is an amazing creation and that it is designed with a built in "blueprint" if given the opportunity, it will heal and repair itself. As a very famous Naturopathic doctor and Master herbalist, Dr. John Christopher, stated:

"There is no such thing as an incurable disease, only incurable people".

CHAPTER 19

BONUS SECTION – ANIMAL FIRST-AID
Basic First-Aid For Our Companion Animals

One of the hardest events we may experience is when a loved one, especially, the young and innocent are hurt or become sick due to some injury or accidental ingestion of a toxic substance. All too often this can occur with our animal companions. For many caregivers, this can be a crippling expense as most insurance will not cover other animals and the little one is left without adequate care. This section will briefly cover some of the most common accidents that can occur in the home for our furry/scaly/feathered loved ones and what you may be able to do to help them heal naturally. Please keep in mind that this is not a substitute for qualified veterinarian care and you must use your best judgment for the life of those in your care. We will be coming out with a book in the near future that is entirely dedicated to holistic animal care.

POISONING

One of the most common issues we have seen with our animal companions is poisoning. Most folks are used to hearing about poisoning for dogs occurring through ingestion of anti-freeze left unguarded on the garage floor or by eating chocolate or households chemicals left laying around the house. While sadly, these events do happen, poisonings can also happen from other less well known sources such as snake bites, eating a toxic plant outside or even eating certain toads, for example.

In each of the above cases, one of the commonly affected organs is the liver. We have found if the liver is attended to right away, the chances of the dog or cat surviving rise significantly. The good news is that what is commonly used for humans often works for other animals as well. Mentioned on page

171 of this book is a description of both the use of Milk Thistle and the formula Liver and gallbladder. Since either of these can be used quite liberally it is difficult to overdose your companion. In most cases we would use a dropperfull of either (or both) every half hour to every hour for eight to ten hours until we saw relief. We had a cat once by the name of Wesa (Cherokee for cat) who had eaten an animal toxic to him. By the time we realized what had happened he was already unresponsive and no longer taking food or water. He lay motionless in our arms and would no longer react to us. We took the above mentioned Liver and Gallbladder and gave it to him every half hour by squirting it gently into his mouth. We also did the same with dropperfuls of water during this period to help keep his kidneys flushing. Within about two hours he began to show signs of responding and began to take the medications more readily. Within a short time he was able to stand and had a full recovery.

I have seen cases when the animal's caregivers did not do the above protocol and the animal sadly passed away.

WOUND CARE

Sadly, I have seen too many cases where a dog or cat had sustained a very severe wound and the veterinarian's go to solution was amputation. It is not my place here to try and second guess another doctor's choice of treatments but simply to suggest that there are other alternatives. I have had the opportunity to witness this with a patient of mine who came into the clinic talking about her dog who had a very badly wounded leg and her veterinarian had suggested the leg be amputated due to the nature and severity of the damage. She asked out of desperation if there was an alternative to losing the leg. I told her that while I could not counter what the vet had stated as the dog was not a patient of mine I did tell her what I had seen in the past with other animals. She was familiar with the Formula called B, F and C, as shown on page 162. This particular case was also mentioned there.

Below is an example of the leg as it healed. Be aware they are quite graphic.

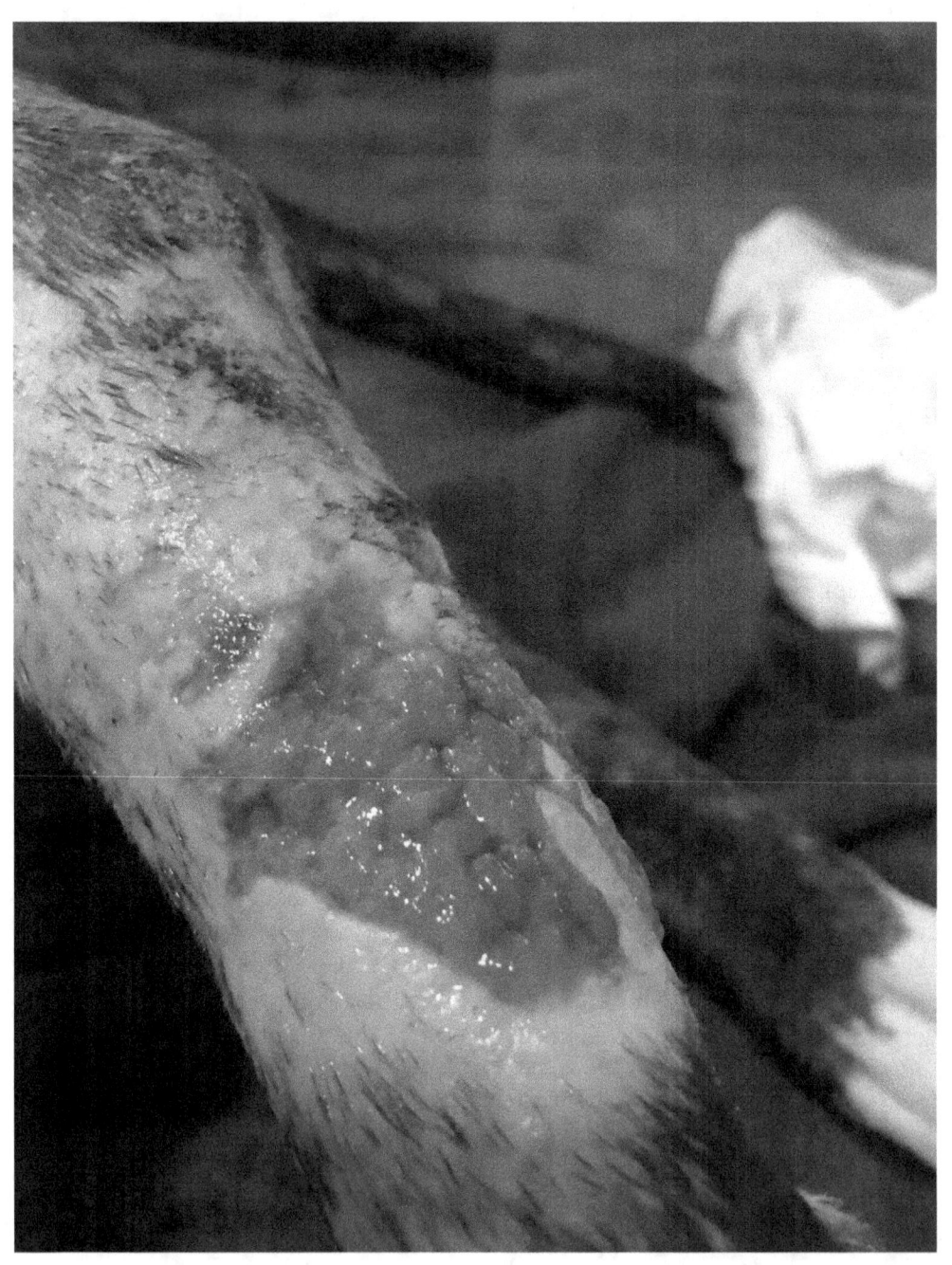

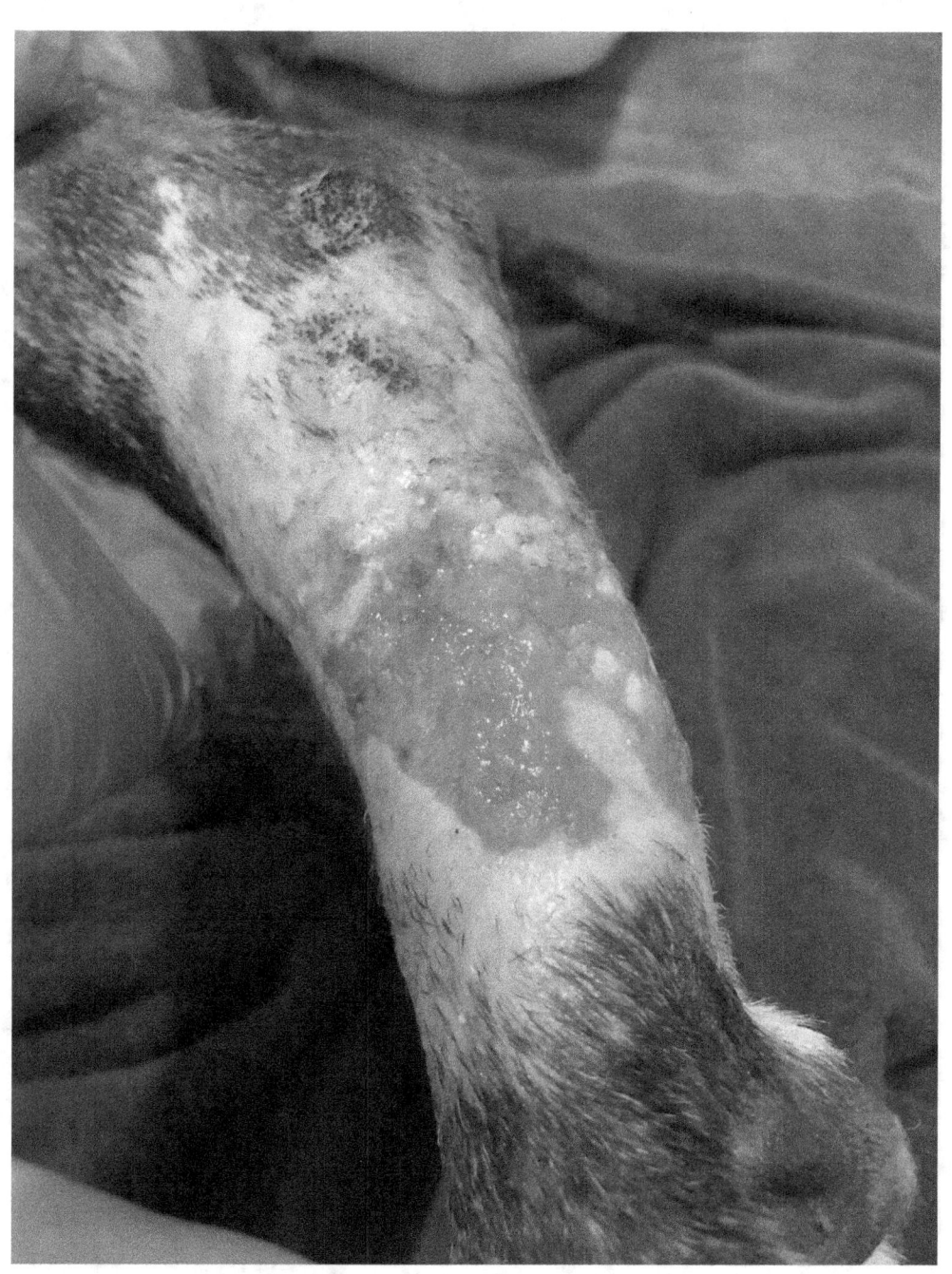

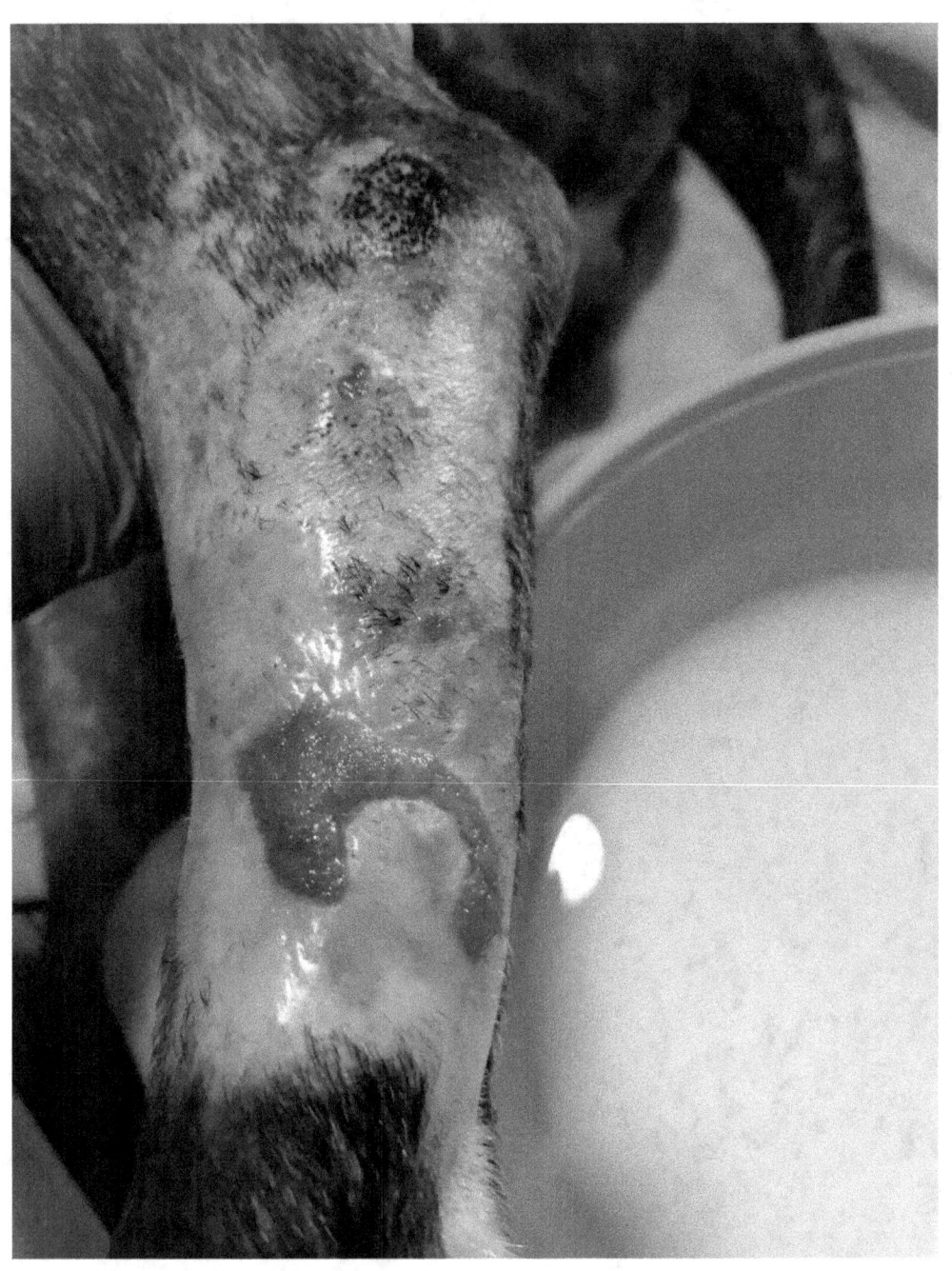

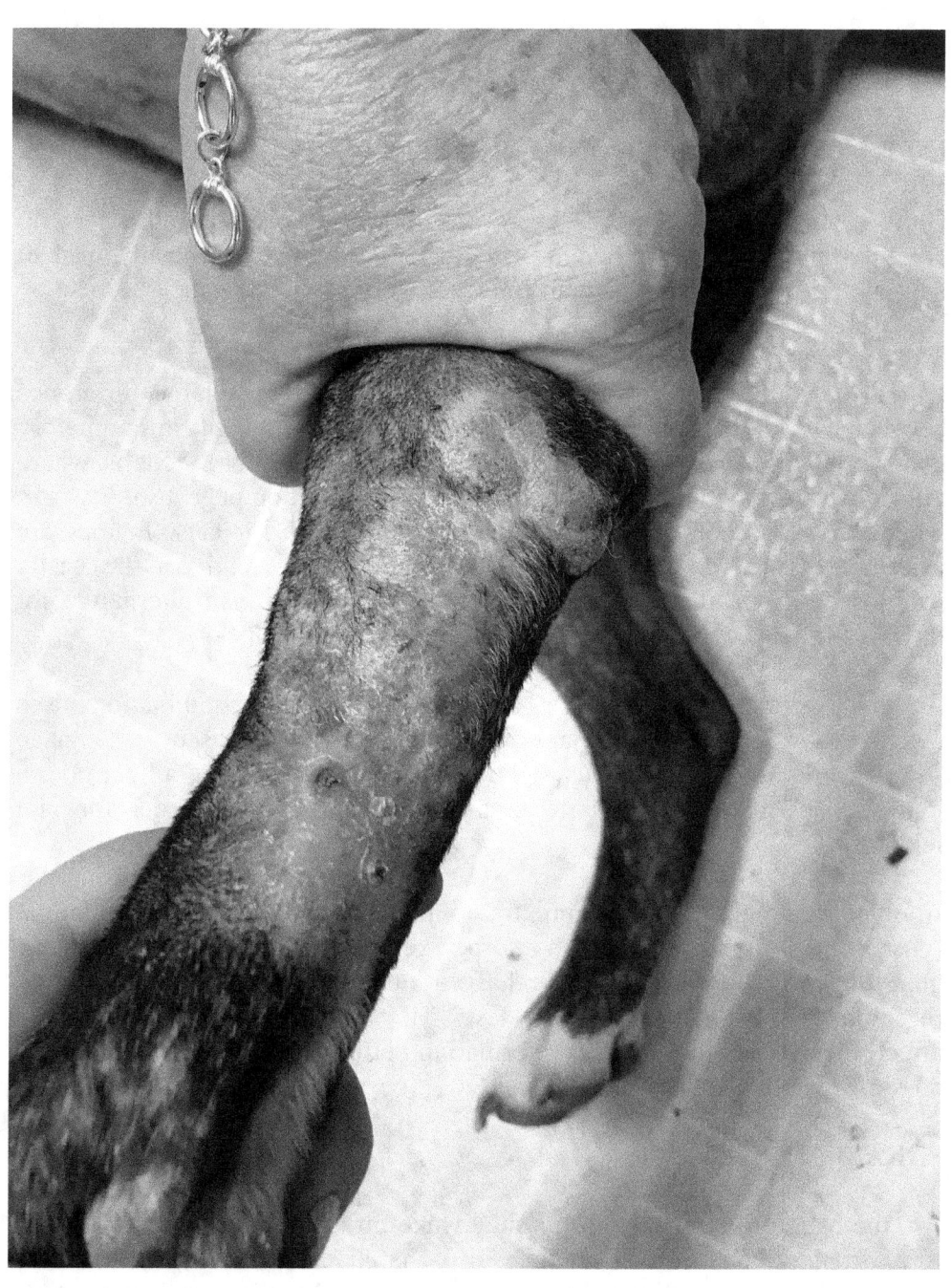

As you can see from the above photos, the leg eventually healed completely and the dog happily kept his leg and is doing well to this day.

INFLAMMATION and PAIN MANAGEMENT

Quite often the animal is in severe pain and we need to find a way to comfort them during the healing process. For this we can easily turn to natural anti-inflammatory as pain relievers, very often the same ones use by humans.

In this case one needs to exercise caution as there is a large difference between cats and dogs in this area. One of the best natural anti-inflammatory that we have is the old tried and true Willow (Salilx alba). This is where aspirin was originally derived. It is described in detail on page 186. It works wonderfully for both humans and canines but NOT for cats. Felines are extremely sensitive to salicylates (found in Willow) and can be easily overdosed. It can therefore become very toxic to cats. An alternative for them is Mullein. A nice picture of it can be seen on page 148.

Another wonderful pain killer and muscle relaxer combination used extensively with humans is Cramp bark and Valerian. It is discussed on page 185. It works well for both cats and dogs. Please keep in mind a little goes a long way. I usually use a quarter to a half a dropperful as needed for pain relief.

Another great pain reliever can be found in a high quality CBD formulation. As with many things, caution should be exercised as here again, a little can go a long way. Dogs for example, have a much higher ratio of cannabinoid receptors than humans so it takes less CBD for them to have the desired affect. Please consult a holistic veterinarian before using as the weight of the dog or cat can make a big difference.

PARASITES

Ah, the bane of so many folks as they wake up to find that not only do the furry friends have worms but they also shared them with the rest of the family. I have seen so many patients come into the clinic and swear they have not been exposed to intestinal worms, only to find out their companion animals had them and then shred them as well. This usually happens when the dog or cat sleeps in the same bed as the human caregiver. I had a case one time when a sweet little nine year old girl came into the clinic presenting a vaginal itch. Her parents discovered a very tiny worm. I asked if they had any other animals living with them and they informed me they had recently added a nine week kitten to their family, discovered walking along outside. The little girl let the new family member sleep with her.

I informed them that the worms actually come out at night and this one apparently took a wrong turn and ended up in a most uncomfortable location. We ran stool tests on both the patient and the kitten and both were positive for parasites. Both were put on the parasite program listed in this book (dosages adjusted for weight) and within a couple of weeks they were parasite free. The protocol and medications are described on page 62.

CANCER AND OTHER CHRONIC CONDITIONS

To cover fairly the full range of treating cancer and other chronic conditions is beyond the scope of this book, I wanted to at least touch on the subject to help gives others hope for their companions.

In most cases I have seen the same holistic treatment used for humans work well for other animals such as dogs and cats, horses, etc. The main emphasis is always one encompassing diet, herbs, massages and other protocols.

A wonderful case history involves a little eleven year old Boston Terrier by the name of Lola who is in the care of our son. Originally, she was found to have a spot of cancer on her ear which the vet removed. Within a few months the cancer reappeared and they ended up removing the entire ear. It was around this time they found she had stage 4 breast cancer. It had metastasized throughout her little body. She was given only six months and only if she had chemotherapy.

They had her try one round of chemotherapy and it made her so sick as well as giving her a urinary tract infection. Our son decided that was enough. They are long distance so they gave us a call and asked if we could help. Of course for our little "grandchild" we were more than happy to help.

The first thing recommended was a change to a plant-based whole food diet. This is actually being recommended by more and more vets for dogs as they do very well on a diet of fruits and vegetables. Almost immediately, within a short span of days, her fatigue improved dramatically and she began to act like a puppy again.

We also started her on a series of herbal medications aimed at cleansing the bowels, blood and her liver. We treated the UTI and within a couple of weeks or so it was gone. The kidneys began to show improvement and the blood in her urine disappeared. The largest tumor which was on her throat completely vanished.

It has now been almost six months and she is still improving wonderfully. She only received the first months chemotherapy and never received another. As stated earlier, our son was told that she would need monthly chemotherapy treatments to simply live another six months. I am happy to see our little one still in our lives and doing so well.

About The Author

Dr. Earendil M. Spindelilus D.N.M., M.H., C.R. - Traditional Naturopath, Holistic Practitioner, Clinical Master Herbalist, Certified Nutritionist, Certified Reflexology, Member of Plant Savers of America, Member of American Botanical Council.

I hold a Doctorate degree in Natural Medicine. I have also been a lecturer since 1999. Board Certified Diplomate of Natural Medicine. Member of the American Council of Holistic Medicine.

I have always had a deep and abiding interest in the Plant Kingdom. Even very young I loved the way the herbs held the mystery of healing within them and how I could learn about them. I traveled around the world learning from different cultures their own unique floras and how they incorporated them into their daily lives. With each new herb I learned how special the world is and how Nature supplies us with all we need. In the 1990s I decided to take my education further and enrolled in the School and Natural Healing, the College of Herbal Medicine. I graduated in 1999 with my Master Herbalist. I have also studied with the New Eden School of Natural Medicine where I completed my Doctorate in Natural Medicine. To date, my wife and I have run two medical centers for natural healing. It has always been a great joy meeting with our patients. We are all meant to live a happy, healthy life and when we allow our body to perform it's innate ability to heal itself then this can happen. I am also a past board member of the Reflexology Association of California as well as a published author/writer of numerous holistic books and articles. I am also a past host of a holistic radio show. We currently run a Holistic YouTube channel.

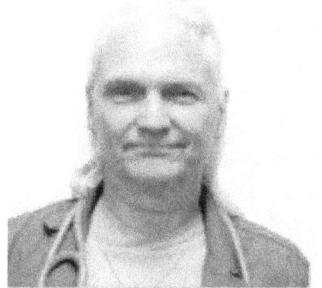

www.ingramcontent.com/pod-product-compliance
Lightning Source LLC
Chambersburg PA
CBHW052341220526
45465CB00003BA/911